The Gerontology Nurse's Guide to the Community-Based Health Network

Brenda L. Bonham Howe, MSN, RN, BSLS, is a nurse educator in the nursing program at Central Oregon Community College, Bend, Oregon. She has worked as a clinical instructor with first- and second-year nursing students. Currently, her main areas of teaching are in the certified nursing assistant program as lecture, lab, and clinical instructor. Ms. Howe believes that a firm foundation in the fundamentals of nursing care results in more holistically cognizant clinical nurses.

Ms. Howe earned a diploma of nursing in 1974 from Legacy Emanuel Hospital's School of Nursing in Portland, Oregon. Twenty years later, she returned to school full time to pursue journalism and research writing. She completed her bachelor of science in liberal studies with the dual minors of social sciences and communication, graduating in 2005 from Eastern Oregon University in La Grande, Oregon. While working toward her BS, Ms. Howe was awarded Outstanding Journalism Student and was recognized among her instructors as a poetry, prose, and fiction writer. In 2002, she earned her master of science as a nurse educator from Gonzaga University in Spokane, Washington.

Her work experience has included rural hospitals and clinics, and a large multispecialty clinic, followed by 7 years of home health and hospice nursing. She piloted and staffed the role of clinical nurse educator in two employment venues, which led to many public speaking engagements. During her home health and hospice work she piloted a foot and nail care clinic for the agency in 2006, which continues to serve hundreds of central Oregon residents. Her work in rural settings, especially as a home health and hospice nurse, inspired her desire to write a guide for nurses to assist clients with navigation of the community health network.

The Gerontology Nurse's Guide to the Community-Based Health Network

Brenda L. Bonham Howe, MSN, RN, BSLS

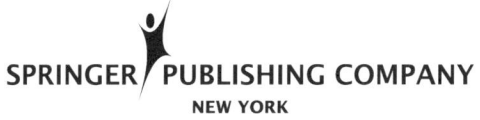

SPRINGER PUBLISHING COMPANY
NEW YORK

Copyright © 2015 Springer Publishing Company, LLC

All rights reserved.

No part of this publication may be reproduced, stored in a retrieval system, or transmitted in any form or by any means, electronic, mechanical, photocopying, recording, or otherwise, without the prior permission of Springer Publishing Company, LLC, or authorization through payment of the appropriate fees to the Copyright Clearance Center, Inc., 222 Rosewood Drive, Danvers, MA 01923, 978-750-8400, fax 978-646-8600, info@copyright.com or on the Web at www.copyright.com.

Springer Publishing Company, LLC
11 West 42nd Street
New York, NY 10036
www.springerpub.com

Acquisitions Editor: Elizabeth Nieginski
Composition: Newgen Knowledge Works

ISBN: 978-0-8261-2701-3
e-book ISBN: 978-0-8261-2702-0

14 15 16 17 / 5 4 3 2 1

The author and the publisher of this Work have made every effort to use sources believed to be reliable to provide information that is accurate and compatible with the standards generally accepted at the time of publication. Because medical science is continually advancing, our knowledge base continues to expand. Therefore, as new information becomes available, changes in procedures become necessary. We recommend that the reader always consult current research and specific institutional policies before performing any clinical procedure. The author and publisher shall not be liable for any special, consequential, or exemplary damages resulting, in whole or in part, from the readers' use of, or reliance on, the information contained in this book. The publisher has no responsibility for the persistence or accuracy of URLs for external or third-party Internet websites referred to in this publication and does not guarantee that any content on such websites is, or will remain, accurate or appropriate.

Library of Congress Cataloging-in-Publication Data

Brenda L. Bonham Howe, author.
  The gerontology nurse's guide to the community-based health network / Brenda L. Bonham Howe.
     p. ; cm.
  Includes bibliographical references and index.
  ISBN 978-0-8261-2701-3 — ISBN 978-0-8261-2702-0 (e-book)
  I. Title.
  [DNLM: 1. Geriatric Nursing--methods. 2. Home Health Nursing—methods. 3. Aged. 4. Clinical Competence. 5. Community Health Services. 6. Health Services for the Aged. WY 152]
  RC954
  618.97'0231--dc23   2014028534

Special discounts on bulk quantities of our books are available to corporations, professional associations, pharmaceutical companies, health care organizations, and other qualifying groups. If you are interested in a custom book, including chapters from more than one of our titles, we can provide that service as well.

For details, please contact:
Special Sales Department, Springer Publishing Company, LLC
11 West 42nd Street, 15th Floor, New York, NY 10036-8002
Phone: 877-687-7476 or 212-431-4370; Fax: 212-941-7842
E-mail: sales@springerpub.com

Printed in the United States of America by McNaughton & Gunn.

*To my parents, Virgil and Inella Bonham,
who inspired me with their stories of surviving
the Great Depression and World War II years.
They remained strong in faith and love
as they grew old gracefully together.
And to my husband, Les,
who encourages me to follow my calling.*

Contents

Contributors   ix

Preface   xi

PART I. GROWING OLD IN THE UNITED STATES

1. Psychosocial–Cultural Health   *1*
   Brenda L. Bonham Howe

2. Health Care Delivery: Cultural Considerations   *11*
   Brenda L. Bonham Howe

3. Health Care Delivery: Cultural Domains   *21*
   Brenda L. Bonham Howe, Maria Milagros Kneusel,
   and Jane A. Tiedt

PART II. PHYSICAL AND PSYCHOLOGICAL CHANGES OF AGING

4. Theoretical Perspectives on Aging and
   Physical Changes   *57*
   Jane A. Tiedt

5. How to Deal With Compromised Independence   *77*
   Brenda L. Bonham Howe

PART III. THE COMMUNITY-BASED HEALTH NETWORK

6. Home-Style Adult Safety and Socialization Options   *97*
   Brenda L. Bonham Howe

7. Home Health Services   *111*
   Brenda L. Bonham Howe

8. Skilled Nurse Competency Requirements for Home Health Services   *179*
   Brenda L. Bonham Howe

9. Hospice and Palliative Care Services   *199*
   Stephanie Bernahl Barss

10. Skilled Nurse Competency Requirements for Hospice Services   *211*
    Brenda L. Bonham Howe

11. Independent Living   *217*
    Brenda L. Bonham Howe

12. Assisted Living   *227*
    Brenda L. Bonham Howe

13. Long-Term Care   *241*
    Kaye Conrath

14. Alzheimer's and Memory Care   *247*
    Brenda L. Bonham Howe

15. Additional Community Health Resources for the Financially Compromised   *255*
    Brenda L. Bonham Howe

PART IV. EMPOWERING THE INNER ADVOCATE

16. Why Must Clients and Caregivers Embrace Self-Advocacy?   *261*
    Brenda L. Bonham Howe and Esther Freeman

Index   *287*

Contributors

Stephanie Bernahl Barss, FNP, MS, RN, CWOCN
Advance Practice Nurse
Partners in Care, Home Health and Hospice
Bend, Oregon

Kaye Conrath, MSN, RN
Adjunct Professor
Resource Center Specialist
Department of Nursing
Gonzaga University
Spokane, Washington

Esther Freeman, MS, CTRS, CPRP
Retired
Tacoma, Washington

Brenda L. Bonham Howe, MSN, RN, BSLS
Nurse Educator
Central Oregon Community College
Bend, Oregon

Maria Milagros Kneusel, MSN, RN
Clinical Instructor
Visiting Nurses Association of Colorado
Bloomfield, Colorado

Jane A. Ticdt, PhD, RN, CDE
Assistant Professor
Department of Nursing
Gonzaga University
Spokane, Washington

Preface

Many times in my career, I have been the nurse at a loss; not knowing where or how to direct a client toward community resources. I recall my own nursing instructors (40 years ago) saying, "You don't need to know all the answers; you need to know where to find the answers you do not possess." The paradox is that novice and experienced nurses must have some leads about how to navigate the unfamiliar community health network. Finding those leads can take up restricted clinical time.

After many years of work in a rural hospital, small medical clinics, and a large multispecialty clinic, I accepted a job in a home health and hospice setting. In the home health venue, my understanding of how community health services network most effectively finally solidified. When that ah-ha moment arrived, memories of various situations gone wrong started to filter through my thoughts. Now I understood how things fall through the cracks because of poor communication or simple lack of understanding about what services are actually available from community health resources. I became increasingly aware that many geriatric clients and their family members are inadequately informed about potential community resources. Providing the information should not be left just to the primary care provider. Now, more than ever, health care professionals must be mindful of their geriatric clients and caregivers and be ready to suggest a direction for them to find the support they need for their journey.

This book is divided into four parts. Part I, "Growing Old in the United States," provides an overview of psychosocial–cultural health and the potential financial and mental drain that occurs when an aging family member loses independence. Potential barriers to health care access are discussed for vulnerable populations. My work in the home health and hospice venue brought me into the midst of functional and dysfunctional family situations where emotions and behaviors reflected the strain of finances, unemployment, substance abuse, language barriers, and folk culture. All of these factors influenced the outcomes of my attempt to promote traditional health precepts. I feel it is vital to possess an understanding of how diversity of culture influences perception of health and illness. Without respect, we will not be as successful in health promotion as we will be in laying another brick in the wall of distance and distrust.

Part II offers insight into a variety of theories about the physical and psychological changes of aging. The information progresses from the physical and physiological changes, to the signs and symptoms that reveal the approach of physical and mental decline. The information provided in Part III provides key information about assistance and living options found in the community when decline is evident. Various optional living situations are described, including how much supportive care is actually provided by the facility or community.

"Empowering the Inner Advocate" is the title of Part IV. As I have visited geriatric clients in many levels of optional living, I have found that having luxury architecture and interior design is not important if the resident-to-caregiver ratio is such that personal hygiene, hydration, nutrition, and socialization are lacking. The mission statement may sound compassionate, but the bottom line may take precedence over the quality of services. It is vital that all advocates for the geriatric population (family and caregivers) continue to speak up, write letters to elected representatives, and promote quality care above profit.

Each chapter in this book, plus the chapter appendices, offers information and links to additional useful resources that are available to the nurse to assist clients in the community-based health network. Many chapters end with a list of topics and references to pertinent websites. A short list of useful key words following the web address represents tabs found on the website home page. When those tabs are selected by the reader, resource links will appear on screen.

It is my hope that the information provided in this book will serve as a valuable tool and source of empowerment for any nurses or support staff who work with the vulnerable geriatric population.

Brenda L. Bonham Howe

1

Psychosocial–Cultural Health

Brenda L. Bonham Howe

SMALLER WORLD, INCREASING LIFE SPAN

Signal change is all around us. Mass media and rapid transit surpass former hurdles of time and space, alerting the world to the constant forces that drive change in every aspect of our lives. It is no surprise to anyone working in health care that we have a growing population of geriatric residents according to census reports (U.S. Census Bureau, 2011). What is alarming are the actual statistics when brought down to the level of our own community, neighborhood, and family circle.

According to the 2011 census, 4.7% of the population was age 65 years and older as compared to 2.8% in 1980. The estimation, based on current relevant statistics (age, gender, health statistics, etc.), predicts that by 2050, this segment of the population will comprise a 10% wedge of the pie graph.

It is known that the longer a person lives, the likelihood of developing a disability increases as does the possibility of living in a long-term care facility. The potential loss of independence is discussed in Chapter 5. Several age-related changes lead to compromised independence. The census report indicates that 98.2% of people in their 90s living in long-term care facilities have one or more disabilities; 80.8% not living in long-term care facilities also had one or more disabilities, usually related to mobility activities. Challenges with mobility are a strong indication that some amount of daily in-home assistance would be required to promote a safer environment (U.S. Census Bureau, 2011).

NONMEDICAL CAREGIVERS

The majority of people requiring long-term assistance receive it in a home setting from a family member or friend. Bodenheimer and Grumbach (2009) state that "twenty-eight million people are informal caregivers." They went on to say in 1996 that these caregivers provided more than $200 billion in unpaid labor. Without a sufficient number of family caregivers, who will pick up the expense of housing or provision of in-home care for the increasing number of geriatric clients? Options for living are discussed in later chapters of this book.

PSYCHOSOCIAL IMPACT

The psychosocial impact is significant as many caregivers must reduce work hours or leave jobs in order to provide necessary care for a family member, because they cannot afford the monthly expense of a facility. Nearly one half of nonmedical caregivers are age 65 years or older and many of them live at the poverty line and often are not in good health themselves (Bodenheimer & Grumbach, 2009). In addition, we live in a country where so many families live miles or states apart. The decision to care for aging parents often means relocating them from the place that is most familiar to them. It is like pulling a mature plant from settled ground. Even healthy plants experience transition shock; why would we expect anything different from an emotional being, even if there is some memory impairment present?

We often refer to the "grief process" or the stages of dying as applied to the loss of a friend, family, or a cherished pet. But the stages of grief may also be viewed as emotional responses to change. Personal construct psychology (PCP) speculates that "how we interact with others is the result of our past experiences and an assessment of the current situation that is then mapped onto possible alternative courses of action." We then choose the course of action that we think will best suit our needs. We may arrive at the conclusion that our behaviors are fluid and shift according to the current situation (Fisher, 2012).

When the time comes for family members to make decisions about living arrangements for their geriatric family members, it triggers the stress hormones ("fight or flight") and our bodies prepare for a very difficult conversation when retreating would be preferred. Even in the most cordial of family groups, to have another family member move into the primary home may eventually generate discord and additional stress. It is not uncommon for family members to still have unsolved childhood issues with the parent(s) or siblings. Each person in the dynamic circle may experience anxiety, anger, dependence, resentment, and depression. Sometimes, that will feel like a vicious cycle; like a tire spinning in sand.

GROWING OLD IS NOT FOR THE FAINT OF HEART—NOR IS BEING A CAREGIVER

Additional factors that increase the burden of care were experienced by the author in the late 1990s. Her father in law lived in a handicapped-accessible studio apartment attached to the main home. The crux of his medical needs included slowly progressing Parkinson's disease, impaired gait, hypertension, being recently widowed (married for 50 years), low back pain syndrome, agitation, and early signs of paranoia. This is one of millions of examples, and much less complex than many other caregivers experience. Although many good memories were made, his unwillingness to comply with use of mobility devices, the risk and experience of his falls, and loss of driver's license (huge loss of independence) increased over a 2-year period. Suspicious of plots against him (his hearing was so bad that he thought his family was whispering about him), complaints about meals not to his "meat and potato" satisfaction, and other undesirable behavior contributed to an emotional drain, even for a trained health care professional with spouse support.

HOME TO COMMUNITY

Years of work as a home health and hospice nurse brought the author into many situations in which family members were involved in the care of an older sibling, parent, or parents. Even in the most loving and supportive home environment, care of another person who has some level of health debility changes the dynamic of life for each member in the circle. Many times, the one needing assistance does not "see" that need as intently as the caregiver. Often, a crisis must occur (a fall and rehabilitation) before an independent-minded geriatric individual will admit to needing some assistance. The culture in the United States is about youthfulness.

This author has questioned many geriatric clients about how old they feel in their head when they think about themselves. Eighty-five-year-old Maxine (fictitious) said, "I think I'm still 17. Yes, that's just how I feel. I feel young in my mind like I did when I left home and started out to make my own way in the world." When gray-haired Rose (fictitious) with senile dementia was asked what she liked to do for fun, she smiled and said, "Oh, I like to chase boys." The shriveled little grandma in the wheelchair next to Rose grinned and said, "Oh, so you like to chase the young ones, do you?" Rose said, "Oh, yes, it can be a lot of fun, but I don't kiss and tell." Others have said, "I think I'm pretty young until I pass a mirror and it's kind of a shock as to who that old woman is."

Stories about geriatric gentlemen seen up on their roof, cleaning their chimney, have been heard more than once (father-in-law included). There are also those lovely silver-haired ladies who climb up on a chair to dust the top of the refrigerator, or reach to change a lightbulb. Until they fall and break something, they "don't want to bother anyone." Recognition of how the body has betrayed their abilities is somewhat blinded by the young thoughts in their head. Family or friends who catch these geriatric "gymnasts" are alerted that mom or dad is no longer able to make safe decisions about what he or she believes he or she is capable of doing alone. The safety factor is often the first "caution" sign to go up. Then, more challenges begin with regard to what to do when independence is compromised.

MENTAL HEALTH AND CAREGIVING

According to the Centers for Disease Control and Prevention (CDC, 2011), mental health problems exist for a larger percentage of disability than any other group of illnesses, including cancer and cardiovascular diseases. Population surveys include measures of mental illness, associated risks (e.g., alcohol consumption and drug abuse), and chronic conditions with related care and clinical services. Two thirds of people in skilled care facilities have a mental illness. Family caregivers are at increased risk of developing mental health problems, if they do not already experience symptoms related to their own situational stress and/or chronic health conditions.

The American Psychiatric Association (APA) speculates more than 65 million family caregivers assist family or friends who need support with activities of daily living (ADL). Those who are caregivers for family members or friends with mental illnesses need support and encouragement just as much as those caring for loved ones with other illnesses.

Caregivers tend to be selfless, and often push themselves beyond their physical and emotional energy levels without recognizing their own need for self-care. Studies demonstrate that caregivers have higher levels of depression and stress than noncaregivers. Sometimes caregivers are so committed to helping others that they forget to take care of themselves. Nurses are notorious for giving until they burn out. Caregivers have a drive to help others, but often fail to recognize that if they drive themselves to exhaustion or sickness, they may not survive for the individuals under their care (APA, 2014). Caregiver burnout is discussed in Chapter 16. Too often, this is a very difficult transition for all involved. As the aging population grows, more nurses should be able to offer information and support to family and potential caregivers. It is vital that current and future nurses become more informed about what is available in the community health network.

NURSING SHORTAGE

An additional challenge associated with the growing proportion of geriatric clients is the fact that 45% of working nurses are aged 45 to 54 years (American Nurses Association [ANA], 2008). The average age of employed registered nurses is 45.5 years. The projected nurse shortage by 2025 is 260,000. How will health care facilities retain adequate, qualified staff to provide care for the complex health needs of the aging population? What will the quality of care be at that time, when we already know that quality of care falls short in many facilities?

> Americans spend twice as much as residents of other developed countries on healthcare, but get lower quality, less efficiency and have the least equitable system...The lower the performance score for equity, the lower the performance on other measures. This suggests that, when a country fails to meet the needs of the most vulnerable, it also fails to meet the needs of the average citizen. (Fox, 2010)

Prior to the 1990s, immigrating nurses trained abroad did not exceed 4,000 a year. President George W. Bush signed a bill in 2005 to release 50,000 visas that brought an upsurge of registered nurses from the Philippines, India, and China. Williams suggests that the import of foreign-educated nurses to help offset the nursing shortage has the potential to mask other problems in the homeland and the work destination (Williams, 2014).

SUMMARY

- Statistics show the increasing population of geriatric citizens.
- The longer individuals live, the higher is the risk of disability and need for assistance.
- As caregivers also age, the financial burden of care may fall on the government, already in financial debt.
- Nonmedically trained caregivers provide more assistance to family or friends than health care facilities combined.
- There are many psychosocial and financial implications for families who have an aging parent or relative who is no longer safe to live independently.
- Aging is a stressful transition as is becoming a caregiver for a family member or friend.
- Current trends for cutting health care costs include moving a significant amount of health care provision from the hospital and back into the community. The need for caregivers in the community is on the rise.
- Mental health issues must be considered when contemplating the dynamics of caregiver and recipient. Priorities must shift for each person, sometimes meaning giving up a job, coping with less income, and losing independence for the geriatric family member. Stress precipitates the fight or flight response, affecting hormone changes and initiating an array of emotional responses that can contribute to the interpersonal dynamics at home.
- The shortage of nurses adds to the concern of who will care for the aging population.

- The following chapters introduce some of the community-based options for assisting both clients and caregivers.

RESOURCES

Astor, B. (2011). *Baby boomer's guide to taking care of aging parents.* Raleigh, NC: Lulu Press.

Konigsberg, R. D. (2012). *The truth about grief. Grieving process—challenging the five stages.* Retrieved May 29, 2014, from http://thetruthaboutgrief.com

National Institute on Aging. (2011). *Why population aging matters: A global perspective.* Corpus Christi, TX: 1001 Property Solutions LLC.

Minority Nurse

Caring for our aging population. Retrieved from http://www.minoritynurse.com/article/caring-our-aging-population

Search Terms
- Caring for our aging population
- Generational schism
- Minority nurses

Nurse Zone

They're not getting any younger: Caring for an aging population. Retrieved from http://www.nursezone.com/Nursing-News-Events/more-features/They%E2%80%99re-Not-Getting-Any-Younger-Caring-for-an-Aging-Population_35022.aspx

Search Terms
- More time to treat
- More Medicare issues
- Age specific concerns

Nurses for a Healthier Tomorrow

Facts about the nursing shortage. Retrieved from http://www.nursesource.org/facts_shortage.html

Search Terms
- Underlying causes
- Frequently asked questions about the nursing shortage

USA Today: Aging Population a Boon for Health Care Workers

Aging population a boon for health care workers. Retrieved from http://www.usatoday.com/story/money/business/2012/10/02/healthcare-job-growth/1600255

Search Terms
- Baby boomers
- Hospital need for nurses
- Home health

REFERENCES

American Nurses Association (ANA). (2008). *Fact sheet: Nursing by the numbers.* Retrieved May 29, 2014, from http://www.nursingworld.org/NursingbytheNumbersFactSheet.aspx

American Psychiatric Association (APA). (2014). *Caregivers—family caregivers.* Retrieved May 29, 2014, from http://www.psychiatry.org/mental-health/people/caregivers

Bodenheimer, T., & Grumbach, K. (2009). *Understanding health policy: A clinical approach* (5th ed., p. 142). New York, NY: McGraw-Hill Medical.

Centers for Disease Control and Prevention (CDC). (2011). *Morbidity and mortality weekly report (MMWR).* September 2, 2011/60(3), 1–32. Retrieved May 29, 2014, from http://www.cdc.gov/mmwr/preview/mmwrhtml/su6003a1.htm

Fisher, J. (2012). *Personal transition curve—the stages of personal change—and introduction to personal construct psychology.* Retrieved May 29, 2014, from www.businessballs.com/personalchangeprocess.htm#personal construct psychology

Fox, M. (2010). *U.S. scored dead last again in healthcare study.* Reuters Edition, U.S. June 6, 2010. Retrieved May 29, 2014, from http://www.reuters.com/article/2010/06/23/us-usa-healthcare-last-idUSTRE65M0SU20100623

U.S. Census Bureau. (2011). *Census bureau releases comprehensive analysis of fast-growing 90-and-older population.* Retrieved May 27, 2014, from http://www.census.gov/newsroom/releases/archives/aging_population/cb11–194.html

Williams, J. (2014). Implication of foreign-educated nurses on United States nursing collegiality. *R.N. Journal.* Retrieved May 29, 2014, from http://rnjournal.com/journal-of-nursing/implication-of-foreign-educated-nurses-on-united-states-nursing-collegiality

2

Health Care Delivery: Cultural Considerations

Brenda L. Bonham Howe

MINORITY GROWTH

Michael Cooper's (2012) *New York Times* article projects the need for the term "minority" in the United States to become obsolete within a few years. According to the U.S. Census Bureau, no single racial or ethnic group will constitute a majority of children older than 18 years by the end of this decade. Within three decades, no single group will exist that is a majority in the United States. The 2010 census indicates a growing population where the elderly make up an increasing portion of the populace, which is evolving in racial and ethnic diversity. The definition of culture developed by the Office of Minority Health (OMH, 2013) incorporates many central themes. It defines culture as "the thoughts, communications, actions, customs, beliefs, values and institutions of racial, ethnic, religious, or social groups." Ethnicity is defined by the OMH as "a group of people that share a common and distinctive racial, national, religious, linguistic, or cultural heritage" (Spector, 2004).

NATIONAL CULTURALLY AND LINGUISTICALLY APPROPRIATE SERVICES STANDARDS

The National Standards for Culturally and Linguistically Appropriate Services (CLAS) in Health and Health Care (known as the National CLAS Standards) went through a formal, 2-year review process and an enhanced version was re-released in April 2013. National CLAS Standards are intended to advance health equity, improve quality, and help eliminate health care disparities by establishing a blueprint for organizations to deliver effective, understandable, and respectful services at every point of patient contact. This program is scheduled to be under annual review for accreditation purposes (U.S. Department of Health and Human Services [USDHHS], 2012).

CLAS outlines steps of governance, leadership, and workforce for the purpose of recruitment, promotion, and support of response to the population within each service area. Those initial leaders, who initiated the standards in a new community service area, strive to educate and train the next level of leadership in the philosophy of CLAS (USDHHS, 2012).

Engagement of like-minded individuals, continuous improvement, and accountability are necessary for the success of CLAS. Appropriate goals must be set, policies developed, and management accountability must be present. Collection of reliable data is important to monitor and evaluate the impact of CLAS (USDHHS, 2012).

INTERPRETER VALIDATION

Language assistance is a key factor in the provision of effective communication with clients. Tools for success include language assistance at no cost to the clients. The interpretive service is advertised on signs or posters (in the preferred language of the clients) and in verbal explanations. Individuals who serve as interpreters must provide legal documentation that validates competence in English and the optional language(s). PSI Services, LLC, has provided certification testing services to more than 60 professional associations over the past years. They maintain an excellent reputation for well-formatted testing criteria to validate an exceptional level of competition. PSI is recognized by the National Board of Certification for Medical Interpreters (NBCMI), launched in 2010 in support of the National CLAS Standards (Langdon, 2010).

Enterprising individuals have seen the growing need for supply of interpreters as a business opportunity. The Yellow Pages and Internet links include listings of agencies that recruit work assignments for interpreters. It is important for customers to validate the qualifications of any potential employee who is a third party in the business arrangements. Training validation may be available in the form of a certificate from a specific training program (i.e., through a community college). Making inquiries about the interpreter's training is important. The ultimate standard is held by the expectations of the NBCMI (Langdon, 2010). Membership in the International Medical Interpreters Association (IMIA, 2014) or the National Council on Interpreting in Health Care (NCIHC, 2014) provides participants a quality of professionalism in addition to opportunities for continuing education, participation in policy development, and advocacy for interpreter and client (IMIA, 2010).

HEALTH CARE CONFLICT

Several variables exist that may provoke conflict from individual members of minority groups when presented with Western medical philosophy: decade of birth, generation in the United States, class, language, and education. Life experiences vary depending on the decade born and the cultural values and norms of the time. Worldviews differ considerably between the immigrant generation and generations to follow. Social class registers higher within some cultures than others (and may be influenced by prior experience or level of education). For example, many foreign born are employed in service industries, skilled work, farms, and manual labor.

Language is a primary factor to consider when inspecting potential sources of conflict in communication. Special needs exist for individuals who cannot hear (or hear well), cannot communicate verbally (use sign language), and do not speak English well or at all. Impediments to successful communication can provoke frustration for both parties and may contribute to cultural and social misunderstandings. This alone may foster mistrust of Western medicine and those who attempt health care delivery (Spector, 2004).

PSYCHOSOCIAL BARRIERS TO SUCCESSFUL HEALTH CARE DELIVERY

Racher and Annis (2007) present *prejudice* as "a deep and visceral dislike of those whose appearances or customs threaten the status quo." Variations of prejudice based on fear of others may be demonstrated in acts of superiority or inferiority. *Ethnocentrism* is the view through the lens of one's personal cultural perspective (normal and preferred). This view filters perceptions through personal values and the belief that the familiar cultural group is superior. When intolerance is demonstrated, tolerance and respect may serve to bridge the gap in communication. Stereotyping is an oversimplification of a plethora of complex layers of information about any one group of people. Stereotypical beliefs may be based on irrelevant information. For example, a family that recently arrived from Ukraine may find American apple pie too sweet or tart. To assume no one from Ukraine will like apple pie is a much generalized assumption. It is important to remember that not all Americans of European descent like apple pie. Stereotyping may precipitate discriminatory practice.

RACISM

No racial group of people adheres to the same cultural beliefs and practices. It is often one's race that precipitates *stereotyping* a group of people. It is possible that racism is an ethical problem where inadequate respect, violation of personal boundaries, and a disparity of power exist (Burkhardt & Nathaniel, 2008). *Discrimination* is exposed when people or groups of people are denied equality of treatment based on their race, ethnicity, age, gender, or disability. In fact, discrimination is the behavioral equivalent of prejudice (Racher & Annis, 2007).

HEALTH CARE ACCESS

Problems of equal health care access are often cited as evidence of racial bias within the American health care system. As the national population has continued to expand in diversity, traditional solutions to health problems are not always planned to meet the education and health promotion programs for minority groups. This is often demonstrated by poorer health outcomes and higher mortality rate (Burkhardt & Nathaniel, 2008).

ETHICAL RESPONSIBILITIES

How do nurses share in the ethical responsibility of promoting health care access and equality? First, review *The International Council of Nurses Code of Ethics 2012* (ICNC). Where inequality exists, it may feel like a "mountain" of complex issues amid a political tug of war over policy and implementation (International Council of Nurses, 2012). By staying in touch with current affairs related to health care delivery, health care professionals are able to self-reflect about personal values and how those may be expressed to bring about change.

Organizational awareness is important; so it is vital that individual employees investigate their employers' policies and actions that represent respect and tolerance for the diversity of employees and clients (Gurchiek, 2008). Then look to the community to consider the diverse population and the dynamics represented in the social and professional groups that make up the local population. There are many avenues of opportunity for professionals and volunteers to help redefine the "mountain" into small, manageable portions. For example, many cities and towns have a community clinic that is supported in part by grants, volunteer health professionals, and donations. These clinics provide an opportunity for people who have no medical insurance to be examined by a doctor, physician assistant, or nurse practitioner. Services are further improved by prescription discount coupons or access to free medication direct from manufacturers. Chapter 15 provides more information about community resources and volunteer opportunities.

SUMMARY

- The need for the term "minority" will one day be obsolete as demonstrated by U.S. Census Bureau statistics.
- National Standards for CLAS in Health and Health Care are intended to advance health equity, improve quality, and help eliminate health care disparities.
- Standards are set to validate and certify medical interpreters.
- Variables exist that contribute to health care conflict: psychosocial barriers, racism, and health care access.
- Nurses share the ethical responsibility of promoting health care access and equality.

RESOURCES

Diversity Statistics in the United States

http://www.stat.purdue.edu/about_us/diversity.html
Black Cultural Center: http://www.purdue.edu/bcc
Diversity Resource Office: http://www.purdue.edu/vpsa/phonefaxdir/pfddive.php
International Center: http://www.intlctr.org
International Students and Scholars Office: http://www.iss.purdue.edu

Latino Cultural Center: http://www.purdue.edu/lcc
Native American Educational and Cultural Center: http://www.purdue.edu/naecc
Office of Institutional Equity (OIE): http://www.purdue.edu
Treasurer's Diversity Task Force: http://www.purdue.edu/treasurer/diversity
Women's Resource Office: http://www.purdue.edu/butler

Search Terms
- Racial and ethnic diversity
- Full-story link

Human Rights Campaign (HRC)

HRC blog. Retrieved from http://www.hrc.org/blog/entry/lgbt-ally-angelina-jolie-opens-up-about-proactive-health-decision

Search Terms
- Lesbian, gay, bisexual, and transgender (LGBT)
- Health and aging
- Workplace

International Council of *Nurses Code of Ethics 2012*

The ICN Code of Ethics for Nurses. Retrieved from http://www.icn.ch/images/stories/documents/about/icncode_english.pdf

Search Terms
- Respect for human dignity
- Relationships to patients
- The nature of health problems
- The right to self-determination
- Relationships with colleagues and others

U.S. Diversity County by County

A county-by-county look at diversity. Retrieved from http://usatoday30.usatoday.com/news/nation/census/county-by-county-diversity.htm

Search Terms
- Ethnic population
- Racial population

Write for Access

Language promotes access to diversity. Retrieved from http://writeforaccess.wordpress.com/2014/05/06/language-promotes-access-to-diversity

Search Terms
- Language promotes access to diversity
- Bilingual
- Future oriented

REFERENCES

Burkhardt, M. A., & Nathaniel A. K. (2008). *Ethics & issues in contemporary nursing* (3rd ed., pp. 408–409). Clifton Park, NY: Delmar Cengage Learning.

Cooper, M. (2012). *Census officials, citing increasing diversity, say U.S. will be a "plurality" nation. New York Times*, December 12, 2012. Retrieved May 6, 2014 from http://www.nytimes.com/2012/12/13/us/us-will-have-no-ethnic-majority-census-finds.html?_r=0

Gurchiek, K. (2008). *Stereotyping caregivers can lead to discrimination.* Society for Human Resource Management (SHRM) Publications. Retrieved May 9, 2014, from http://www.shrm.org/Publications/HRNews/Pages/StereotypingCaregiversDiscrimination.aspx

International Council of Nurses. (2012). *The International Council of Nurses Code of Ethics 2012.* Retrieved May 8, 2014, from http://www.icn.ch/images/stories/documents/about/icncode_english.pdf

International Medical Interpreters Association (IMIA). (2014). Retrieved May 5, 2014, from http://www.imiaweb.org/education/LLTesting.asp

Langdon, E. (2010). *First-ever National Medical Interpreter Certification Exams validated and administered by PSI.* National Board of Certification for Medical Interpreters. Retrieved May 6, 2014, from http://www.certifiedmedicalinterpreters.org/national-medical-int

National Council on Interpreting in Health Care (NCIHC). (2014). Retrieved May 6, 2014, from http://www.ncihc.org/organizational-structure

Office of Minority Health (OMH). (2013). *Think cultural health*. U.S. Department of Health & Human Services. Retrieved May 6, 2014, from http://minorityhealth.hhs.gov/templates/browse.aspx?lvl=2&lvlID=15

Racher, F. E., & Annis, R. C. (2007). Respecting culture and honoring diversity in community practice. *Research and Theory for Nursing Practice: An International Journal, 21*(4). Spring Publishing Company. Retrieved May 8, 2014, from http://web.b.ebscohost.com.proxy.foley.gonzaga.edu/ehost/pdfviewer/pdfviewer?vid=3&sid=171bf0e4-ed0a-492f-aeeb-c485ead2586b%40sessionmgr110&hid=120

Spector, R. E. (2004). *Cultural diversity in health and illness*. Upper Saddle River, NJ: Pearson Prentice Hall.

3

Health Care Delivery: Cultural Domains

Brenda L. Bonham Howe, Maria Milagros Kneusel, and Jane A. Tiedt

The purpose of this chapter is to encourage the reader to consider his or her own cultural identity and heritage. Furthermore, the reader needs to think about biases and stereotypes that may exist in his or her own perspectives. Generalization is a simplistic way for our brains to store information (Proenza, 2003). Unfortunately, generalizing falls short of identifying complex traits found in other people. Instead, stereotyping promotes impressions that lead to judgment and misunderstanding. For example, what comes to mind when you read the following phrases?

- The _____ love to drink beer, but the _____ love their whiskey and the _____ prefer wine.
- The _____ love their watermelon.
- _____ eat beans for breakfast, lunch, and dinner.
- _____ eat raw fish and rice.

Did you first think of one cultural or ethnic group of people to associate with the food or beverage? We may instantly associate one cultural group with each food or beverage, but in fact, many people from all cultural groups partake of the items listed. Our immediate response reflects assumptions learned from childhood, from people around us, and the media.

In order to develop an awareness and understanding of how complex the issues of modern health care delivery are, it is important to self-reflect and develop an awareness of how we perceive how others respond to us. We are complex as individuals, but the interactions that occur in our network of family, friends, casual acquaintances, and so on, create multiple layers and patterns in our thinking and behavior. Those we network with are just as complex. This is one reason why, as nurses, we must respect and promote respect as directed by our conscience and *The International Council of Nurses' Code of Ethics 2012* (International Council of Nurses [ICN], 2012).

CULTURAL DOMAIN

National Standards for Culturally and Linguistically Appropriate Services in Health and Health Care (National CLAS Standards) were discussed in Chapter 2 in addition to some of the barriers to health care delivery systems. It is quite evident that access to health care is a problem for the vulnerable populations in the United States. The reasons for those barriers to health care are varied, and it is important to understand how they came to exist before they can be traversed.

Each person represents the product of a cultural domain. Within each domain is a group of people who identify with a very similar set of values, beliefs, foods, traditional clothing, music, and social practices. How health and illness are perceived is also part of the cultural traditions. For some, illness is an imbalance in the person's body or spirit. Others may believe that a curse has been put on them. The health belief model (HBM) states that individual beliefs affect the actions a person takes relating to his or her health. The HBM was developed by M. H. Becker (1977), a social psychologist in a research project when he was trying to establish why there was a lack of participation by individuals in a free tuberculosis-screening project. The HBM has been modified over time and now contains four variables: perceived susceptibility, perceived severity, thoughts concerning effectiveness of recommended action, and perceived barriers (Rawlett, 2011).

The expectation that every group within multiple domains will assimilate into one culture has not happened in the history of this nation (nor any other for that matter). In order to reduce current barriers to health care access, it is vital that all health care providers begin to appreciate the cultural background of clients (Racher & Annis, 2007). Too often, the casual observer decides that the clients who do not follow the recommended treatment are "noncompliant." Perhaps the real cause is that the information has not been presented in such a way that the client's perceived risk and susceptibility are fully understood. In order to promote self-efficacy, there must be effective communication with apparent proof that the client fully understands. When the client does understand the severity, then recommendations may be discussed to determine if the client is ready to accept the suggestions. If not, further discussion may reveal cultural perceptions that influence the client's willingness to buy into the recommendations. No bridge can be built without the foundation of understanding how Western medicine is perceived by individuals who adhere to a different health care model.

There are several excellent resources available that list cultural groups individually. Rachel Spector (2004) is a noted author on the subject of cultural diversity and health care. Many books and articles are attributed to her and may be found online. The Stanford School of Medicine offers a geriatric education website that includes extensive information about ethnogeriatric competencies (sgec .stanford.edu). It would take a book of encyclopedic proportion to include all of the information that is available.

For the purpose of this chapter, two thorough reviews provide an opportunity for the reader to compare and contrast his or her own perceptions about family, health, illness, and spirituality. Once the examples are read, it is the hope of the authors that some barriers have been minimized.

HEALTH AND ILLNESS IN THE HISPANIC POPULATION

Family Model

The Hispanic or Latino family model is typically a traditional one. Father, mother, and children form the nuclear family unit. Many Hispanics also have larger families, though this is changing with younger generations (Suro, 2007). The nuclear family unit has strong ties to extended family members. Grandparents, aunts, uncles, and cousins are actively engaged in the life of the nuclear family to the point that they are often included in health care decisions.

Hispanics prefer to care for aging parents at home. This is seen as a way of honoring or "paying back" maternal or paternal sacrifices made to provide for children and move the family ahead. If elderly parents are placed in a nursing home, the elderly person may experience a sense of abandonment and become depressed.

In addition to caring for aging parents, Hispanics will often share their homes with adult children and grandchildren. This leads to family units that are multigenerational. Multigenerational family units result in a wide range of health care needs within one household. They also afford patients the benefit of a solid support network (Suro, 2007).

Nurses caring for Hispanic patients can expect to find large numbers of people in the patient's home or hospital room, particularly during a health crisis. It is important for the nurse to identify who the decision maker is among the group and directly communicate with that person, while allowing others to express their concerns and questions.

Gender Role

Gender roles are traditional. The father is the head of the family and often the main provider, decision maker, and protector. Hispanic fathers are strongly involved in the rearing of their children, both female and male. Typically, the role of the father is that of passing on character traits such as work ethics, respect for others, and the promotion of education, while mothers become more engaged in teaching social graces and religious beliefs (Cabrera & Tamis-LeMonda, 2013). Older male children may become the decision makers if the father is not present or able to make decisions. Women working outside the home is commonplace, especially among younger generations, and for many immigrant families.

Religious or Spiritual Needs

The majority (68%) of Hispanics in the United States identify themselves as Catholics. The next largest denomination among Hispanics is Evangelical Protestants with 15% of Hispanics in the United States identifying themselves as such (The Pew Forum on Religion and Public Life [PRC], 2007). Some speculate that the election of the first Hispanic Pope in April 2013 will cause an increase in the number of Hispanics who identify themselves as Catholics.

Catholicism

The Catholic tradition has a long history in Hispanic life. In early colonial times, Catholic missionaries from Europe became actively engaged in the work of spreading the Catholic faith throughout Central and South America. One of the events that was most influential in cementing the Catholic tradition among Hispanics was the apparition of Our Lady of Guadalupe, which took place in Mexico in the year 1531 (Figure 3.1). Any nurse who is caring for Hispanic Catholics should be familiar with this event.

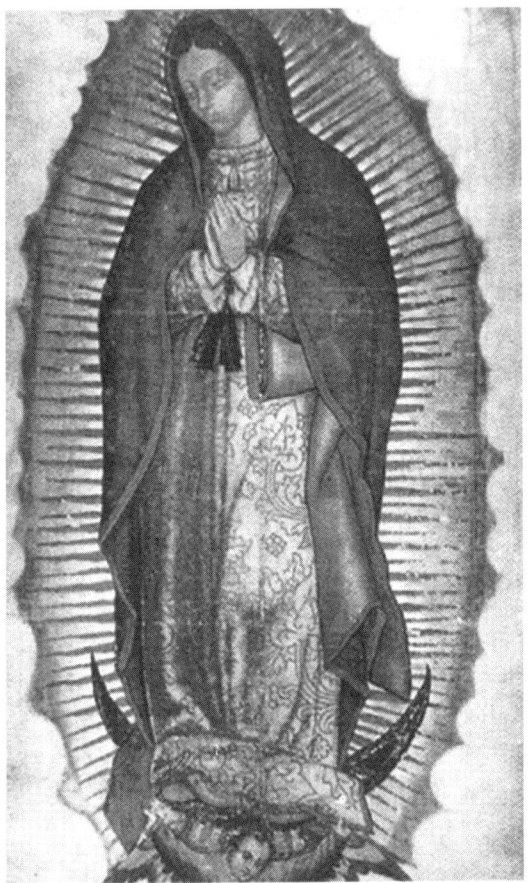

FIGURE 3.1 Our Lady of Guadalupe in a facsimile of a 15th-century engraving.

The story is as follows: The Virgin Mary, the mother of Jesus and a central figure in Catholicism, appeared to a poor native man named Juan Diego. The Virgin asked Juan Diego to go to the bishop and request that a chapel be built to honor her visit. Juan Diego's story was accepted by the bishop when an image of the Virgin miraculously appeared on Juan Diego's *tilma*, a type of apron worn by natives. The Virgin was given the title of Our Lady of Guadalupe and the chapel was built. The chapel is now known as the Basilica of Our Lady of Guadalupe and it houses Juan Diego's tilma, which still bears the miraculous image. The basilica is an important place of worship where many Hispanics go to seek miracles, particularly healing from physical ailments. Nurses who care for Hispanic patients can expect to see images of Our Lady of Guadalupe carried by family members or posted near the patient's bed.

The Catholic faith is rich in symbols, traditions, and liturgical practices. Nurses caring for Hispanic Catholics may see them use *sacramentals*, items that, when used as intended by the church, help to increase the believer's devotion and inclination to virtue (Tonnes, 1950).

One sacramental commonly used by Hispanics is a *scapular*. A scapular is a small piece of brown cloth with a holy image usually worn around the neck. The scapular is particularly valued when a patient is near death, since Catholics believe that those who die reverently wearing it are spared the fires of hell. If the patient is unable to wear the scapular, it is sufficient to have it on him or her.

Hispanic Catholic patients will also require the use of *sacraments*. Sacraments are different from sacramentals in that they are actions or events through which the person can receive divine grace. There are seven sacraments in the Catholic church and some are not optional for those who actively practice their Catholicism. Sacraments that are particularly sought by patients during the time of illness are: Reconciliation, Eucharist, and Anointing of the Sick.

Reconciliation is also known as confession. This sacrament can only be administered by a Catholic priest. During reconciliation, the penitent (patient) will tell his or her sins to the priest who will then administer the sacrament, thereby absolving or forgiving the penitent's sins. If the patient requesting reconciliation is Spanish only, it would be important to find a priest who can speak Spanish. Reconciliation may be sought before any procedure where there is risk of death, such as surgery.

Eucharist is also known as *Communion*. During Communion, the Catholic patient is given sacred bread to eat. Receiving Communion is considered the height of the Catholic–Christian experience because Catholics consider this sacred bread to be, in fact, the body of Jesus Christ. Eucharistic bread wafers are therefore to be treated with the utmost reverence and respect. Many Hispanics avoid receiving or asking for this sacrament because they often feel unworthy to receive it. The nurse may still ask the patient if he or she wishes to receive the Eucharist.

Finally, Anointing of the Sick is a sacrament that involves ritual prayers as well as the use of holy oils. This sacrament can only be administered by a Catholic priest and is given to persons who are seriously ill or in danger of death. It was formerly known as Extreme Unction. Catholics believe that the Anointing of the Sick always heals the soul in preparation for death, and sometimes the body as well.

Evangelical Protestantism

Evangelical Protestantism, the second largest religious affiliation among Hispanics in the United States, is a Christian denomination. Evangelical Protestants base their faith in the Bible. Nurses caring for Evangelical Hispanics should make a bible available to them. If the patient is Spanish only, a Spanish-language bible should be obtained.

When it comes to health, Evangelicals believe in the healing power of Jesus, who is God. The healing power of Jesus is made available to persons who are ill through prayers of petition offered privately by the sick person or through the intercessory prayers of fellow Christians. Intercessory prayer is based on the belief that God's actions may be influenced by the petitioner or intercessor and result in a change in nature and world events. This belief is rooted in biblical principles, particularly the example and teachings of Jesus who performed miraculous healings and assured his followers of the power of intercessory prayer (Elwell, 1996). When engaging in intercessory prayer, the petitioner or intercessor will ask God to supply healing and restore the sick person to health. Intercessory prayer may be done quietly or loudly and can include the "laying on of hands" (touching the sick person). During prayer, the intercessors may sing and lift their hands in a gesture of petition. The nurse should be aware that Evangelical Hispanics are likely to practice the laying on of hands during intercessory prayer, and provide any necessary instructions warranted by the patient's condition, such as an explanation of contact precautions.

In addition to intercessory prayer, fellowship with church members is very important to Evangelical Protestants and a vital source of consolation and support for the patient. Whenever possible, the patient should be allowed visits from church members.

Regardless of what specific religion is practiced, Hispanics are people strongly influenced by faith in God and belief in the supernatural. They use spiritual practices that engage the senses and emotions. Illnesses may be viewed as the result of lack of faith and devotion, or attributed to the effects of curses. Hispanic patients and their families readily ask for God's help in times of illness or while grieving, and expect miracles. Leaving things *en las manos de Dios* (in God's hands) is a common attitude. The nurse who cares for Hispanic patients must be competent in issues related to spirituality.

Attitudes About Health Care and Health Issues

Respeto

A significant attitude toward health and health care, found among Hispanics, is that of *respeto* (respect). Hispanic persons are taught from a young age to show proper respect to persons in authority. To show *respeto*, Hispanic persons adopt a submissive attitude, limit direct eye contact and verbal interactions, and avoid speech that may seem confrontational or questioning. They may only speak when spoken to. Because doctors and nurses are seen as authority figures, Hispanic patients tend to display these actions when receiving health care. This may cause communication gaps between patient and provider and diminish the quality of care given to the Hispanic patient. Nurses caring for Hispanic patients can encourage openness by asking friendly questions about family and other topics of interest before asking about the patient's condition. This type of "small talk" can create a climate of trust and lead the patient to share more information when health care needs are addressed (Purnell & Paulanka, 2008). The nurse should give patients ample time to answer questions, because Hispanic patients like to share their experiences in detail and usually begin by providing all of the background information they find relevant to their current situation.

Indigenous/Folk Healing Practices

Even though the overwhelming majority (87%) of Hispanics in the United States prefer Western medicine, there are a number of Hispanics who believe in using indigenous/folk healing practices such as *Santeria* or *Curanderismo* (Livingston, Minushkin, & Cohn, 2008).

Santeria is commonly practiced by Caribbean Hispanics such as Cubans or Dominicans. It is based on religious beliefs brought to the islands by African slaves. Santeria involves the actions of a practitioner, a *santero*, who serves as a diviner or fortune-teller as well as an intermediary between the client and a variety of deities. These deities, also known as *orichas*, rule over the different parts of the body. The illness of a particular body part is often seen as a punishment for wrongdoing against the deity who rules that body part. During Santeria rituals, these deities use the santero to communicate healing remedies that may include the use of herbs, specific incantations, and animal sacrifices. The deities of Santeria are represented by images or statues, which are sometimes borrowed from Catholicism (Chevannes, 2013).

Curanderismo, which means "curing works," is a system of healing practices that stem from an assortment of sources including European witchcraft, ancient humoral pathology, Native American lore, Judeo–Christian rituals, and psychic phenomena. Curanderismo is practiced by healers known as *curanderos*. Curanderos declare healing powers in three areas: spiritual, mental, and material. Curanderos who claim spiritual healing powers function as mediums between the patient and *corrientes espirituales* (spiritual currents), which are said to guide the patient's healing process. Mental healing powers involve the ability of the curandero to manipulate his or her mental energy and direct it to the patient's healing. Material powers involve the use of objects and substances such as amulets or herbs along with certain rituals to rid the patient of illness or the effects of some other negative event (Cavender, Gonzales Galdson, Cummings, & Hammet, 2011).

It should be pointed out that Catholicism and Evangelical Protestantism forbid the use of healing practices they attribute to the occult, including Santeria and Curanderismo. This can cause conflict among Hispanic family members.

Privacy

While Hispanics are friendly and open in their communications with one another, there are topics that they consider personal and private.

As a general rule, it is considered rude to ask a Hispanic person about his or her financial situation or salary. If a nurse or health care worker needs to inquire about the patient's ability to pay for services, it should be done in private and tactfully, explaining why the information is necessary.

Discussions about sexual topics are also considered private. When discussing sexual matters or dealing with reproductive health issues, Hispanic patients, especially those from older generations, prefer to talk to someone of their same gender. In addition, sexual topics should not be discussed in mixed company. Some married couples may openly discuss sexual issues among themselves, but this is not necessarily the case. The nurse should inquire about the couple's views on discussing these issues together.

Issues that occur between family members, such as disagreements regarding end-of-life (EOL) care, are considered private. Because of the strong family ties, Hispanic people resent outsiders who interpose their views or act as if they have equal status to a family member. Private family matters may be discussed with close friends, but Hispanic patients do not share family issues with strangers (Martinez-Houben, 2012). Health care providers need to establish a rapport with the patient and family before they are able to provide appropriate care.

Food

Another item worth mentioning is the importance of food in the Hispanic culture. Eating is an important bonding experience, which is central to the development and strengthening of relationships. Eating alone is seen as a negative experience. In addition, Hispanic families love to prepare and share food and become concerned when a person looks *muy flaco* (too skinny). Eating more is often seen as a solution to illness. Hispanics tend to eat only a light breakfast, with lunch being the largest meal of the day. Unless they have adopted North American schedules, Hispanics tend to eat dinner late in the evening (Purnell & Paulanka, 2008).

Potential Problems and Solutions

Language Barriers

The first obvious issue many Hispanic patients face when seeking health care in the United States is a language barrier. The native language of most Hispanics is Spanish. While some Hispanics, such as Puerto Ricans, are bilingual, immigrants from other Hispanic countries may not speak English. To breach this gap in communication, the U.S. Department of Health and Human Services (USDHHS) has developed national standards for the provision of CLAS. These standards should be used by nurses caring for Hispanic patients who have a language barrier (USDHHS, n.d.). CLAS standards can be accessed at www.thinkculturalhealth.hhs.gov/pdfs/EnhancedNationalCLASStandards.pdf.

Lack of Primary Health Care Providers

Many Hispanic patients do not have a main or primary health care provider. When asked why in a recent survey, the majority of respondents (41%) stated that they do not get sick often enough to warrant having a primary provider. Seventeen percent stated that they lack a primary provider because they do not have health insurance and 13% stated that they prefer to treat themselves (Livingston et al., 2008).

Nurses should be aware of this trend among Hispanic patients as it will impact discharge planning and follow-up of medical conditions. The lack of primary health care providers is particularly concerning because four out of the five leading causes of death among Hispanics are chronic illnesses that require significant management. These are cancer, heart disease, unintentional injuries, stroke, and diabetes (Centers for Disease Control and Prevention [CDC], 2013).

Obtaining Health Care Information

According to the CDC, Hispanic patients receive most of their health care information via TV and radio. They are particularly attentive to messages spread through Spanish-speaking TV and radio celebrities. In addition, Hispanics respond well to health care information that is given to them by other members of their community. Various efforts aimed at increasing patient knowledge of conditions like diabetes have proved that establishing *promotoras* in the community works well. Promotoras are health advisers who work individually with patients in their homes or community centers. Promotoras teach and explain issues related to healthy living (CDC, n.d.).

The Hispanic culture is complex and each individual expresses his or her Latino heritage in unique ways. The information just presented here will be helpful for the nurse who wishes to provide culturally competent care.

HEALTH AND ILLNESS IN THE NATIVE AMERICAN POPULATION

There are more than 500 federally recognized Native American tribes in the United States each with its own distinct values, language, and history (Figure 3.2). When working with Native American people, it is important to avoid stereotyping or generalizing. There are similarities in tribes living in close geographic proximity; there can also be significant differences. Tribes from the Pacific Northwest or Plains states have very distinct beliefs, practices, and traditions that may not be the same as those of tribes from the Eastern or Southern United States. The terms American Indians or Native Americans are often used synonymously. They refer to people indigenous to North America. There is no correct definition, but many prefer their original tribal or clan name: Nimipuu instead of Nez Perce or Dine instead of Navajo, for example. The terms American Indian and Alaska Native (AI/AN) are federal government constructs for record-keeping purposes. Of the 562 federally recognized tribes, more than 200 are Alaska Native villages and the rest are located in 33 other states (Fleming, 1995).

According to the 2010 U.S. census, there are 5.2 million people who self-identify as AI/AN either alone or in combination with other racial or ethnic groups. The population continued to grow by 18% per the 2000 census and by 27% per the 2010 census. The states

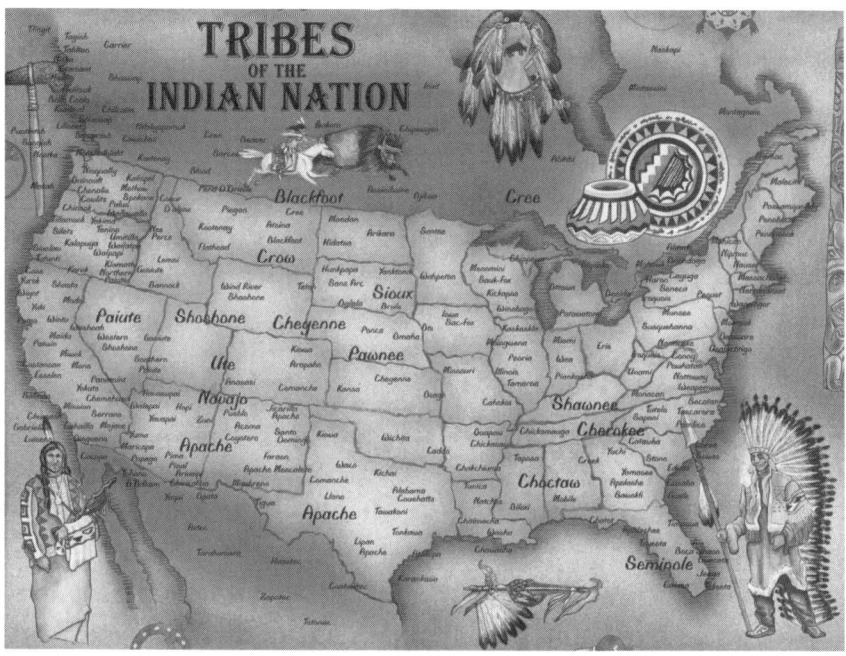

FIGURE 3.2 A map depicting the locations of American Native tribes.

with the highest numbers of Native American people are California, Oklahoma, Arizona, Texas, New York, New Mexico, Washington, Florida, and Michigan. Two thirds of the Native American populations live outside of tribal areas. Less than one quarter live on reservations or trust lands. The largest tribes in the United States are the Cherokee, Navajo, Choctaw, Chippewa, Sioux, Apache, Blackfeet, and Creek (Norris, Vines, & Hoeffel, 2012).

Historical Background

To better understand the Native American people, one must first be aware of some of the legal and historical background between the U.S. government and tribes as they have evolved over the centuries. In exchange for tribal lands and compensation for relocation to reservations, various treaties and laws were established to protect and support the Native American people (Schmidt, 2011).

Treaty Period

Since 1778, the U.S. government negotiated treaty relationships with Native American tribes, which obligate the federal government to uphold tribal sovereignty; safeguard Indian trust property; and provide medical, educational, and social services for the health and welfare of Native American people. The U.S. Constitution recognizes tribes as sovereign nations established through government-to-government treaty relationships. Tribal sovereignty means that each tribe has the right to self-govern and the right to negotiate with the government as an independent nation. Tribal sovereignty was upheld by the Supreme Court in the 1830s and has been the foundation for numerous statutes, and judicial and administrative rulings (Morrison, Fox, Cross, & Paul, 2010).

Reservation Period

As American settlers moved westward, reservations began to mark the western landscape (Trennert, 1998). The Indian Removal Act (1830) forced more than 100,000 Native Americans from their homelands in the eastern United States to reservations west of the Mississippi River. Thousands of Native American people died in the process. With greater numbers of tribal people living on reservation lands, the U.S. government had to address the growing problem of illness and disease. Due to confinement on the reservation and poor sanitation conditions, infectious diseases were rampant, resulting in a catastrophic decline in the Native American population (Shoemaker, 1999).

For tribes located near military forts, Army doctors did take steps to curb these epidemics (Shelton, 2001). In 1849, the Bureau of Indian Affairs (BIA) was charged with overseeing Native American health care (Rhoades, 2000). In 1873, the BIA created the Medical and Education Division. The responsibilities of the Medical branch were liquor control, sanitation, and improving the health and welfare of the Native American people. The leading diseases on the reservations were pneumonia, syphilis, rheumatism, consumption, and smallpox. A smallpox vaccine program was their first large public health campaign, due in large part to fear of the smallpox epidemic spreading to the White population (Trennert, 1998). Unfortunately, most efforts of the Medical and Education Division were made toward the civilization of the Native Americans and medical care remained inadequate (Rhoades, 2000).

Assimilation and Allotment Period

The next phase of government action was assimilation and allotment (Shelton, 2001). Missionary crusades were supported in an effort to assimilate the Native American people through education and Christianity. Many Christian missionaries and educators believed that the Native American people were doomed to extinction unless they were civilized and assimilated into the dominant society. The government paid subsidies to the missionary churches to educate the Native American children. Tribal youth were forced to attend boarding schools away from home. They were given Anglo-Saxon clothing and haircuts and given Christian names. The children were also not allowed to see their families or speak their native language. On reservations, traditional spiritual and healing practices were prohibited. Violations resulted in jail time or loss of monthly food provisions (Shelton, 2001; Wilkinson, 2005).

With the insidious western expansion, the Dawes Allotment Act of 1887 was enacted. The reservation lands were broken up into parcels. The head male in each Native American household was given an allotment of reservation land and taught to farm it. The goal was for each family to be self-supporting. However, few tribal members were interested in farming or giving up their traditional ways of hunting, fishing, and doing seasonal rounds. Land ownership was the antithesis to their belief system; so many families lost their parcel to greedy landowners or to the government for taxes owed. More than 90 million acres of reservation land was ceded to the government and opened up to mining, logging, and farming interests by the time the Dawes Act was repealed in 1934 (Shelton, 2001; Wilkinson, 2005).

Conditions on the reservations remained harsh. With no hospitals and few physicians, the BIA began hiring field matrons, often from missionary organizations, to provide some health care services to tribal members living in remote areas. These women provided basic medical care and education on nutrition, food preparation, sanitation practices, and prenatal care (Trennert, 1998). By the early 1900s, the government began to realize the full devastation of health care problems on the reservations. Epidemics of tuberculosis (TB) and trachoma were problematic, especially in the close confines of boarding schools. The 1928 Merriam report was highly critical of the U.S. government's failure to provide adequate funding for health care services and described the dismal failure of the assimilation and allotment programs. Efforts to correct the situation were met with strong political resistance (Shelton, 2001).

Congress transferred Indian health care services and facilities to the Public Health Service (PHS) in 1954 because health care services were so inadequate under the BIA. The agency was renamed Indian Health Services (IHS). IHS secured funds to promote highly qualified medical staff, update facilities, improve sanitation conditions, and establish prevention programs (Rhoades, 2000).

Termination Period

During the 1940s and 1950s, a federal termination policy was enacted to eliminate treaty responsibilities with tribes by forcing total assimilation. This process involved the sale of tribal land, termination of sovereign nation status, and imposing state and federal jurisdiction (Shelton, 2001). Native Americans from terminated tribes were relocated to urban areas where jobs were more plentiful. The intent was that they would receive job training and seek employment. Between 1952 and 1972, approximately 100,000 Native Americans from 60 tribes were relocated to cities (Snipp, 2000). They were ill prepared; so many of the relocated families just ended up on welfare rolls (Roubideaux, 2005). The effects of termination were devastating to the health and welfare of tribal communities and Native American people (Shelton, 2001).

Self-Determination Period

In a move toward self-determination, President Nixon reaffirmed the treaty commitment, calling for the federal repeal of the termination policy. He also recommended granting tribal control and management of federal Indian health programs. As a result, the Indian Self-Determination and Education Assistance Act (PL 93–638) was passed into law in 1975 (Kickingbird & Rhoades, 2000). In 1976, the Indian Health Care Improvement Act was passed. This mandated specific IHS health benefits including inpatient and outpatient care; dental, mental-health, and addiction counseling; and preventive services. The goal was to eliminate health disparities and promote self-determination by allowing tribes to control and manage their own programs (Rhoades, 2000).

Title I of PL 93–638 offers tribes the choice of managing their own health care programs. They can contract with IHS for the health services. After 3 years of successful contracting with IHS, tribes are eligible to enter into a self-governance contract with IHS. This gives the tribe the flexibility to allocate resources and design programs without having to go through the federal bureaucracy (Dixon, Mather, Shelton, & Roubideaux, 2001).

IHS remains perpetually underfunded and understaffed (Roubideaux, 2005). The current IHS budget only provides 59% of funding needed to provide basic health care services. According to a report by the U.S. Commission on Civil Rights (USCCR, 2003), the federal government has budgeted almost twice as much per capita for health care to federal prisoners than is funded per capita to IHS for Indian health. For the USDHHS, Native American health remains a low priority, with IHS accounting for only 0.5% of the total USDHHS budget (USCCR, 2003).

Indian Health Services

The USDHHS oversees IHS. The IHS headquarters are located in Rockville, Maryland. There are 12 regional offices: Aberdeen, Alaska; Albuquerque, New Mexico; Bemidji, Minnesota; Billings, Montana; throughout California; Nashville, Tennessee; the Navajo area; Oklahoma City, Oklahoma; Phoenix, Arizona; Portland, Oregon; and Tucson, Arizona. The regional offices oversee medical facilities and services. IHS provides health care services to approximately 57% of Native Americans who are members of federally recognized tribes and live within the IHS service area. IHS runs 33 hospitals, 55 clinics, and 38 health centers. Through Public Law 93–638 contracts, IHS provides cooperative management of 15 hospitals, 229 health centers, 116 health stations, and 116 Alaska village clinics. The challenge for IHS is to remain financially solvent while addressing the growing burden of managing chronic diseases (Rhoades, 2000).

IHS also subsidizes 41 urban Native American programs throughout the United States. As predominantly referral centers, these sites provided 700,000 service visits to 1.3 million Native Americans residing in urban areas (Northwest Portland Area Indian Health Board [NPAIHB], 2007). With more than half the Native American population residing in urban areas, access to health care is an ongoing challenge (Sherwood, Harnack, & Story, 2000).

For those who qualify, IHS services are provided at no charge (Dixon, 2001). To be eligible for services, one must be a Native American, a member of a federally recognized tribe, and living within the IHS service area for that tribe. Tribal members living at a distance from their own reservation do not qualify for IHS services. Furthermore, IHS does not provide funding for them to obtain care where they do reside (Rhoades, 2000). Tribal members must live in the service area for at least 180 days before they can qualify for IHS care. They must obtain preapproval for referrals to specialists or hospital care outside of IHS. If allotted funds for IHS are used for the fiscal year, they must wait until the next fiscal year to get approval for the service (Dixon, 2001).

Health Care Needs

Early Health Concerns

Native Americans' health concerns prior to Columbus included infectious diseases, traumatic injuries, and malnutrition. The arrival of Europeans to North America brought a host of diseases including smallpox, diphtheria, chicken pox, mumps, measles, typhoid, and influenza, to which the Native Americans had no acquired immunity (Jones, 2004). Their health declined dramatically after tribes were confined to reservations. Until the mid-20th century, Native Americans experienced higher morbidity and mortality rates than the general U.S. population because of poor sanitation and inadequate health care. When IHS became a part of the PHS in the 1950s, conditions on the reservations were ameliorated. Since then, decreasing infectious disease rates have been replaced by an epidemic of chronic diseases (Trennert, 1998).

Shifting to Chronic Diseases

The greatest concern for the health and welfare of Native Americans in the 21st century is the disproportionate burden of chronic illnesses. The origins are rooted in social and ecological issues including poverty, living conditions, discrimination, cultural barriers, and access to care (Tashiro, 2005). A study comparing utilization and access to health care for Native Americans found that Native Americans had limited insurance or access to health care and less utilization of services than Whites (Zuckerman, Haley, Roubideaux, & Lillie-Blanton, 2004). Although IHS does provide some care to those living in service areas, access remains limited. In addition, those with IHS care receive less preventive care than the White population (Zuckerman et al., 2004). Overall, the health care for Native Americans has improved since the 1950s. However, they still have a lower life expectancy than Whites, Latinos, or Asian Americans (Olshansky et al., 2012).

Beliefs and Values

Each tribe has its own unique set of values and beliefs. There are some common patterns, although these are not universal. The first is the belief in one supreme creator. This higher power is often referred to as Great Spirit, Creator, or Great One. Second, there is a strong connection with nature; all things are interrelated. Plants, animals, minerals, and humans are all a part of the world as it was created and they are all intricately intertwined together. What happens to one affects the others. The earth is sacred and there is oneness among all living things. The Native American people are very careful about how they treat all living things because all are connected (Portman & Garrett, 2006).

In the Native American culture, family and community are very important. A strong bond to family, clan, community, tribe, and land provides a sense of belonging. This kinship bond involves extended family and can include nonrelatives as well. In many tribes, there is no distinction between married or blood relatives; they are all family. The concept of family is more in alignment with the traditional notion of an extended family rather than a nuclear family; often multiple generations live together in one household. Care of children is shared among family members and many aunts, uncles, and grandparents help in the child-rearing process. There is a great love for children (Deacon,

Pendley, Hinson, & Hinson, 2011). In addition, elders and women are honored and respected. Gender roles tend to be balanced. Men and women have varying responsibilities depending on the tribe.

A sense of community permeates all aspects of their lives, which promotes a sense of unity, cooperation, and cohesion. The needs of the larger family or community take precedence over individual wishes. This is reflected in their community orientation to care and support others. Sharing and gift giving are common. The underlying premise is that if one has more than one needs, one gives it away. Giving demonstrates honor and respect (Lettenberger-Klein, Fish, & Hecker, 2013).

Elders play a significant role in tribal communities. They are revered for their wisdom, experience, and the knowledge they have acquired over the years. Elders are treated with deference; so they are asked to speak first or are served first during meals. In meetings or gatherings, it is respectful to allow the elders to lead the discussion without interrupting. The elders offer advice and teaching, often indirectly through storytelling. Depending on the tribe, the term elder refers to those older than 55 years (Hendrix, 2001).

Humor and laughter hold a special place in the everyday lives of the Native American people, especially in the relationships among kin, particularly grandparents and children. The humor is often self-directed. Teasing and jesting are common (Dean, 2003). Native American humor draws on the stories of animal people, especially the trickster coyote. Humor is a critical part of the culture and serves several functions. It is used to demonstrate affection and is a way of paying tribute to another. Humor is a great method to address underlying concerns or to deliver a serious message. The function of humor includes correcting behavior, friendly teasing toward other tribes, relieving stress, or helping to cope with a traumatic event (Gruber, 2008).

In the Native American worldview, things proceed when they are ready to happen. Time is fluid and not structured into linear segments as it occurs in dominant culture. Many Native Americans are present oriented and focus on what they are doing in the moment. This principle stems from a respect for others and being present to the here and now. This takes priority over some future event based on a specific date and time. In the Native American culture, the focus of work is on what is needed for a specific purpose rather than working on a timeline or generating possessions (Twiss, 2000). In general, materialism is not a part of the Native American value system. Accumulating things contradicts their cultural traditions of giving and only taking and using what is needed (Portman & Garrett, 2006).

Communication

Quietness is respected in Native American life and is based in tribal survival. Native people are comfortable with long periods of silence. Do not mistake their silence for ignorance or stoicism. Listening is valued over talking: speaking is from the heart rather than the head. When asked a question, it is respectful to think about how to answer before responding. Expect long pauses in conversation, especially with elders. Make sure not to interrupt when elders speak.

In uncomfortable situations like a medical examination, Native American people may remain silent. It is important to avoid intrusive questions, especially early in the client–clinician encounter. Start with casual conversation to establish rapport. Be open to allowing things to evolve. In patient care situations, it is important not to rush the encounter. For Native Americans, patience is virtue, grounded in the belief that all things will unfold in good time. Patience shows respect for others. It is important to allow time for thoughtful deliberation and even group consensus. Often family members will be involved in patient decision making. Applying pressure toward Native American clients to make quick decisions or responses without deliberation can be detrimental to establishing or maintaining a trust relationship. During client–clinician interactions, it is best to avoid rapid-fire or intrusive questions. Questions should be framed to show respect and caring (Hendrix, 2001).

Nonverbal communication is also important. Native Americans may look down as a sign of respect or deference for someone in a position of authority. Looking down may also show disapproval or dissatisfaction. Avoid direct eye contact or using a loud voice as it may be considered rude. A vigorous, tight handshake may also be considered rude. A light, gentle handshake or touching fingertips is a sign of respect rather than weakness. Be aware of personal space and respect boundaries. Avoid asking too many personal questions too quickly (Dixon & Iron, 2006).

In the Native American culture, information and traditions are passed on through stories rather than through writing. Oral traditions have been passed down since time immemorial. These stories have highly significant meaning for social norms and ethical behaviors. They provide guidance on how to live in harmony with all living things. Storytelling is a way of passing on the tribal history and transmission of the cultural heritage from one generation to the next (Moss et al., 2005; Struthers & Littlejohn, 1999). Use storytelling, pictures, metaphors, and verbal explanations for health education rather than written material when working with Native American clients. Use humor to relieve tensions or break the ice.

Spiritual Beliefs

Spirituality is integrated into the fabric of traditional Native American life. Spirituality is considered a natural element in everything; all living things are connected. Because of that connection, it is important to seek balance between people and the environment. It is a mutual respect, not human domination over the land. The earth is sacred and should be respected and preserved. It is not a resource or commodity for sale. Everything has a place and purpose, so treat the earth with reverence. Maintaining balance and harmony crosses over into spiritual and religious practices. There are still strong religious ties on many reservations depending on which missionary churches were affiliated with the tribe. Native

Americans may be devoted Catholics yet participate in sweat ceremonies and use traditional healers (Twiss, 2000).

The medicine wheel provides the guiding framework for balance and wholeness (Figure 3.3). There are many variations of the medicine wheel among tribes. It symbolizes various cycles of nature and how life is a circular journey. Native American culture is based on a circular way of life. The medicine wheel is divided into quadrants. It symbolizes the four directions, the four seasons, the four stages of life, or the four dimensions of health (Roberts, Harper, Tuttle-Eagle

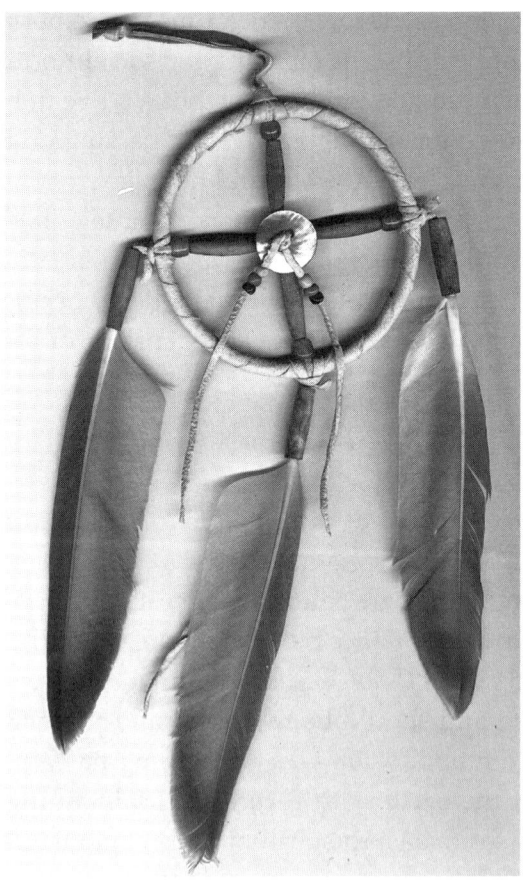

FIGURE 3.3 Medicine wheel of the Lakota Native American people.

Bull, & Heideman-Provost, 1998). It can also represent guiding values. Each section of the circle offers gifts and teachings that can help keep or restore a person's balance (Dapice, 2006). When there is disruption, the four directions need to be realigned in order to walk in balance within the four domains of health: mental, emotional, physical, and spiritual. Otherwise, imbalance can cause discord, stress, and illness (Coyhis & Simonelli, 2005).

Health and Illness

The underlying premise for health and wellness in the Native American culture is to live in harmony so that an individual is in balance with all living things. Humans are made of the mind, body, and spirit. Wellness is achieved when these elements are in balance with one another. In contrast, when there is disharmony among these elements, illness can result. Healing involves restoring harmony with oneself and with one's surroundings. For Native Americans, health and wellness are tied to nature in a holistic fashion (Portman & Garrett, 2006; Rybak & Decker-Fitts, 2009).

Healing Traditions

Traditional healing practices are private. They can be very sacred and may be taboo to discuss them with anyone outside the community. These practices may include herbs, teas, or special foods and may integrate the use of prayers, songs, and ceremonies. Spiritual healers, including medicine men, medicine women, and shamans may perform prayers and healing ceremonies or integrate herbs. These may be used in conjunction with Western allopathic medicine or therapies. Examples of more common traditional rituals include smudging, sweat lodges, and pipe ceremonies (Broome & Broome, 2007; Flowers, 2005; O'Brien, Anslow, Begay, Pereira, & Sullivan, 2002). Smudging is a purification ceremony used to facilitate the healing process. Small amounts of herbs such as sweet grass, sage, cedar, or juniper are burned in an abalone shell to create whiffs of smoke. The smoke is swept over a person, object, or the room. Participants will take the smoke in their hands and wash it over their bodies, especially the area needing healing or cleansing from negative energy (Moghaddam & Momper, 2011).

The sweat lodge is a ceremonial sauna that is used for purification and healing. The sweat lodge and ceremonial sweat vary from tribe to tribe. There are usually two key roles—the sweat lodge leader and the fire keeper. Rocks are heated in a fire outside the lodge. The hot stones are placed in a pit inside the lodge and the door is closed. While participants gather around in a circle inside the sweat lodge, songs and prayers are offered by the leader while herbs and water are sprinkled on the hot rocks. This may be repeated a number of times. The sweat helps reconnect the mind, body, and spirit with Mother Earth. Participation in the sweat lodge is viewed as cleansing and starting life anew. It is akin to rebirth (Portman & Garrett, 2006; Rybak & Decker-Fitts, 2009).

Pipe ceremonies are used to connect the physical and spiritual worlds by carrying prayers to the creator through the smoke. In this ceremony, participants either stand or sit in a circle and pass the pipe from one person to another. Tobacco, kinnickkinnick, red willow bark, or other herbs are used. Participation in ceremonies and rituals helps to restore one to a state of balance (Portman & Garrett, 2006; Rybak & Decker-Fitts, 2009).

Care Considerations

Many Native Americans distrust the health care system. The boarding-school experience left many feeling vulnerable to authority figures. Mistrust is also based on historical trauma from discrimination, exploitation, and forced assimilation (Weaver, 2011). When working with Native American clients, it is important to avoid generalizations and stereotyping. Show respect by asking permission and listening to clients and giving them time to respond.

Sometimes the last thing that's said is the most important. It takes time to establish a trusting relationship; so be patient and demonstrate a caring, casual demeanor (Dixon & Iron, 2006). Be genuine and self-disclosure is appropriate. If you are unsure how to proceed in the client–clinician interaction, just ask. Admit your knowledge limitations and ask the client's guidance to understand the issue and help to create a plan of action together. Frame questions in a way that conveys respect and caring (Hendrix, 2001).

Cultural practices and preferences at the EOL differ widely among tribes and even among individuals within the same tribe. Therefore, it is important to individualize plans of care and avoid making assumptions or generalizations. EOL decisions can be complicated and this is compounded for many Native Americans because of historical experiences of prejudice and exploitation by authority figures (Kitzes & Berger, 2004). Discussions about advance directives can be particularly sensitive. Talking about these issues may be perceived as premature and goes against the orientation that all things happen when they are supposed to. Bringing up death and dying prematurely may cause it to happen. It may be appropriate to provide information on what services are available and ask what they need or how you can assist (Baldridge, 2011).

The long history of discrimination toward Native Americans has created mistrust. Many do not believe that the health care system supports their best interests. They may perceive the provider's discussion about ceasing aggressive treatment or promoting palliative care in place of treatment options as a continuation of discrimination (Zager & Yancy, 2011). EOL care needs to be provided in a manner that does not traumatize the patient or family by institutionalizing a loved one. Provide options for care that are close to nature and family. Try to facilitate cultural practices and personal food preferences, and incorporate traditional healers as desired. Any personal artifacts such as feathers, stones, shells, sweet grass, medicine bags, or religious items should not be touched. These are sacred and highly personal (Castleden, Crooks, Hanlon, & Schuurman, 2010; Flowers, 2005).

SUMMARY

Families may not want to discuss impending death; to speak of it may bring it on prematurely. Mourning for their loved one may not be done openly. The patient may be stoic and not demonstrate pain; so pain management can be challenging. They may not ask for pain medication more than once. Death is a natural part of life that should not be feared. Native Americans rely on their families to carry out EOL wishes when the time comes (Zager & Yancy, 2011).

After death, be sensitive to the family's preferences. The spirit must be whole in order to go into the next world; so many tribes do not support organ donation or autopsy. Some patients may request tissues and organs be returned after surgery so they can be preserved and taken with them into the next life. Speaking the name of the person who has left this world or using the terms dead or deceased is prohibited in some tribes. Doing so may prevent them from transitioning into the spirit world of the ancestors (Hendrix, 2001).

RESOURCES

Health Exchange

www.health-exchange.net/culture.html

Search Terms
- Culture and Health
- Culture Q & A
- Cultural Competence

Transcultural Nursing

www.culturediversity.org/provc.htm

Search Terms
- Beliefs
- Practices
- Habits
- Likes
- Dislikes
- Customs
- Rituals

REFERENCES

Baldridge, D. (2011). Ask a simple question: Four model programs help American Indians plan for end of life. *Aging Today, 32*(6), 12.

Broome, B., & Broome, R. (2007). Native Americans: Traditional healing. *Urological Nursing, 27*(2), 161–163, 173.

Cabrera, N. J., & Tamis-LeMonda, C. S. (Eds.). (2013). *Handbook of father involvement: Multidisciplinary perspectives* (2nd ed.). New York, NY: Routledge.

Castleden, H., Crooks, V. A., Hanlon, N., & Schuurman, N. (2010). Providers' perceptions of Aboriginal palliative care in British Columbia's rural interior. *Health and Social Care in the Community, 18*(5), 483–491. doi: 10.111/j.1365-2524.2010.00922.x

Cavender, A., Gonzales Galdson, V., Cummings, J., & Hammet, M. (2011). Curanderismo in Appalachia: The use of remedios caseros among Latinos in northeastern Tennessee. *Journal of Appalachian Studies, 17*(1/2), 144–167. Retrieved from http://www.jstor.org/stable/41446939

Centers for Disease Control and Prevention (CDC). (2013). *Hispanic-Latino populations*. Retrieved from http://www.cdc.gov/minorityhealth/populations/REMP/hispanic.html#10

Centers for Disease Control and Prevention (CDC). (n.d.). *Building our understanding: Culture insights. Communicating with Hispanic/Latinos*. Retrieved from http://www.cdc.gov/healthycommunitiesprogram/tools/pdf/hispanic_latinos_insight.pdf

Chevannes, B. (2013). *Caribbean healing traditions: Implications for health and mental health*. New York, NY: Routledge

Coyhis, D., & Simonelli, R. (2005). Rebuilding Native American communities. *Child Welfare, 84*(2), 323–368.

Dapice, A. N. (2006). The medicine wheel. *Journal of Transcultural Nursing, 17*(3), 251–260. doi: 10.1177/1043659606288383

Deacon, Z., Pendley, J., Hinson, W. R., & Hinson, J. D. (2011). Chokka-chaffa' kilimpi', chikashshiyaakni' kilimpi': Strong family, strong nation. *American Indian and Alaska Native Mental Health Research, 18*(2), 41–63.

Dean, R. A. (2003). Native American humor: Implications for transcultural nursing. *Journal of Transcultural Nursing, 14*(1), 62–65. doi: 10.1177/1043659602238352

Dixon, M. (2001). Access to care issues for Native American consumers. In M. Dixon & Y. Roubideaux (Eds.), *Promises to keep: Public health policy for American Indians & Alaska Natives in the 21st century* (pp. 61–88). Washington, DC: American Public Health Association.

Dixon, M., & Iron, P. E. (2006). *Strategies for cultural competency in Indian health care*. Washington, DC: American Public Health Association.

Dixon, M., Mather, D. T., Shelton, B. L., & Roubideaux, Y. (2001). Economic and organizational changes in health care systems. In M. Dixon & Y. Roubideaux (Eds.), *Promises to keep: Public health policy for American Indians & Alaska Natives in the 21st century* (pp. 89–121). Washington, DC: American Public Health Association.

Elwell, W. A. (1996). Prayer. In *Baker's evangelical dictionary of biblical theology*. Grand Rapids, MI: Baker Book House Company. Retrieved from http://www.studylight.org/dic/bed/view.cgi?n=563

Fleming, C. M. (1995). American Indians and Alaska Natives: Changing societies past and present. In M. E. Orlandi (Ed.), *Cultural competence for evaluators: A guide for alcohol and other drug abuse prevention practitioners working with ethnic/racial communities* (pp. 147–172). Washington, DC: Department of Health & Human Services (SMA 95–3066).

Flowers, D. L. (2005). Culturally competent nursing care for American Indian clients in a critical care setting. *Critical Care Nurse, 25*(1), 45–50.

Gruber, E. (2008). *Humor in contemporary Native North American literature: Reimagining nativeness*. Rochester, NY: Camden House.

Health and Human Services (HHS). (n.d.). *The national CLAS standards*. Retrieved from http://minorityhealth.hhs.gov/templates/browse.aspx?lvl=2&lvlID=15

Hendrix, L. R. (2001). *Health and healthcare for American Indian and Alaska Native elders*. Retrieved from http://www.stanford.edu/group/ethnoger/americanindian.html

International Council of Nurses (2012). *The International Council of Nurses Code of Ethics 2012*. Retrieved May 8, 2014, from http://www.icn.ch/images/stories/documents/about/icncode_english.pdf

Jones, D. S. (2004). *Rationalizing epidemics: Meanings and uses of American Indian mortality since 1600*. Cambridge, MA: Harvard University Press.

Kickingbird, K., & Rhoades, E. R. (2000). The relation of Indian Nations to the U.S. government. In E. R. Rhoades (Ed.), *American Indian health: Innovations in health care, promotion and policy* (pp. 61–73). Baltimore, MD: Johns Hopkins University Press.

Kitzes, J., & Berger, L. (2004). End-of-life issues for American Indians/Alaska Natives: Insights from one Indian Health Service area. *Journal of Palliative Care, 7*(6), 830–838.

Lettenberger-Klein, C. G., Fish, J. N., & Hecker, L. L. (2013). Cultural competence when working with American Indian populations: A couple and family therapist perspective. *American Journal of Family Therapy, 41*(2), 148–159. doi: 10.1080/01926187.2012.665273

Livingston, G., Minushkin, S., & Cohn, D. (2008). *Hispanics and health care in the United States: Access, information and knowledge*. Washington, DC: Pew Hispanic Center and Robert Wood Johnson Foundation. Retrieved from http://www.pewhispanic.org/files/reports/91.pdf

Martinez-Houben, L. (2012). *Counseling Hispanics through loss, grief and bereavement: A guide for mental health professionals*. New York, NY: Springer.

Moghaddam, J. F., & Momper, S. L. (2011). Integrating spiritual and western treatment modalities in a Native American substance user center: Provider perspectives. *Substance Use and Misuse, 46*(11), 1431–1437. doi: 10.3109/10826084.2011.592441

Morrison, C., Fox, K., Cross, T., & Paul, R., (2010). Permanency through Wabanaki eyes: A narrative perspective from "the people who live where the sun rises." *Child Welfare, 89*(1), 103–123.

Moss, M., Tibbetts, L., Henly, S. J., Dahlen, B. J., Patchell, B., & Struthers, R. (2005). Strengthening American Indian nurse science training through tradition: Partnering with elders. *Journal of Cultural Diversity, 12*(2), 50–55.

Norris, T., Vines, P. L., & Hoeffel, E. M. (2012). *The American Indian and Alaska Native population: 2010 [Census Brief]*. Washington, DC: U.S. Department of Commerce. Retrieved from https://www.census.gov/prod/cen2010/briefs/c2010br-10.pdf

Northwest Portland Area Indian Health Board (NPAIHB). (2007). *NPAIHB policy brief: IHS budget update*. Retrieved from http://www.npaihb.org/policy/policy_briefs

O'Brien, B. L., Anslow, R. M., Begay, W., Pereira, B. A., & Sullivan, M. P. (2002). 21st century rural nursing: Navajo traditional and western medicine. *Nursing Administration Quarterly, 26*(5), 47–57.

Olshansky, S., Antonucci, T., Berkman, L., Binstock, R., Boersch-Supan, A., Cacioppo, J., ... Rowe, J. (2012). Differences in life expectancy due to race and educational differences are widening, and many may not catch up. *Health Affairs, 31*(8), 1803–1813. doi: 10.1377.hlthaff.2011.0746

Pew Forum on Religion and Public Life (PRC). (2007). *Changing faiths: Latinos and the transformation of American religion*. Retrieved from http://www.pewforum.org/files/2007/04/hispanics-religion-07-final-mar08.pdf

Portman, T. A., & Garrett, M. T. (2006). Native American healing traditions. *International Journal of Disability, Development and Education, 53*(4), 453–469. doi: 10.1080/10349120601008647

Proenza, L. (2003). *Stereotypes and generalities*. University of Akron Commencement speech. December 13, 2003. Retrieved May 25, 2014, from http://www.uakron.edu/president/co_12_13_03PM.php

Purnell. L. D., & Paulanka, B. J., (2008). *Transcultural health care: A culturally competent approach* (3rd ed.). Philadelphia, PA: F.A. Davis.

Racher, F. E., & Annis, R. C. (2007). Respecting culture and honoring diversity in community practice. *Research and Theory for Nursing Practice: An International Journal, 21*(4), 255–270. Springer Publishing Company. Retrieved May 8, 2014, from http://web.b.ebscohost.com.proxy.foley.gonzaga.edu/ehost/pdfviewer/pdf viewer?vid=3&sid=171bf0e4-ed0a-492f-aeeb-c485ead2586b%40sessionmgr110&hid=120

Rawlett, K. (2011). Analytical evaluation of the health belief model and the vulnerable populations conceptual model applied to a medically underserved, rural population. *International Journal of Applied Science and Technology, 1*(2), 15–21.

Rhoades, E. R. (Ed.) (2000). *American Indian health: Innovations in health care, promotion, and policy*. Baltimore, MD: Johns Hopkins University Press.

Roberts, R. L., Harper, R., Tuttle-Eagle Bull, D., & Heideman-Provost, L. (1998). The Native American medicine wheel and individual psychology: Common themes. *The Journal of Individual Psychology, 54*(1), 135–145.

Retrieved from http://pzacad.pitzer.edu/~hfairchi/pdf/psychology/Roberts(1998)NativeAmerCounseling.pdf

Roubideaux, Y. (2005). Beyond Red Lake—The persistent crisis in American Indian health care. *New England Journal of Medicine, 353*(18), 1881–1883.

Rybak, C., & Decker-Fitts, A. (2009). Understanding Native American healing practices. *Counseling Psychology Quarterly, 22*(3), 333–342. doi: 10.1080/09515070903270900

Schmidt, R. W. (2011). American Indian identity and blood quantum in the 21st century: A critical review. *Journal of Anthropology, 2011*(549521). doi: 10.1155.2011/549521

Shelton, B. L. (2001). Legal and historical basis of Indian health care. In M. Dixon & Y. Roubideaux (Eds.), *Promises to keep: Public health policy for American Indians & Alaska Natives in the 21st century* (pp. 1–30). Washington, DC: American Public Health Association.

Sherwood, N. E., Harnack, L., & Story, M. (2000). Weight-loss practices, nutrition beliefs, and weight-loss program preferences of urban American Indian women. *Journal of the American Dietetic Association, 100*(4), 442–446.

Shoemaker, N. (1999). *American Indian population: Recovery in the twentieth century.* Albuquerque, NM: University of New Mexico Press.

Snipp, C. M. (2000). Selected demographic characteristics of Indians. In E. R. Rhoades (Ed.), *American Indian health: Innovations in health care, promotion, and policy* (pp. 41–57). Baltimore, MD: Johns Hopkins University Press.

Spector, R. E. (2004). *Cultural diversity in health and illness* (pp. 301–305). Upper Saddle River, NJ: Pearson Prentice Hall.

Struthers, R., & Littlejohn, S. (1999). The essence of Native American nursing. *Journal of Transcultural Nursing, 10*(2), 131–135.

Suro, R. (2007). *The Hispanic family in flux.* Center on Children and Families. Retrieved from http://www.brookings.edu/~/media/research/files/papers/2007/11/hispanicfamily%20suro/11_hispanicfamily_suro.pdf

Tashiro, C. J. (2005). Health disparities in the context of mixed race: Challenges in the ideology of race. *Advances in Nursing Science, 28*(3), 203–211.

Tonnes, A. (1950). *Talks on the sacramentals.* Retrieved from http://www.ewtn.com/library/LITURGY/TLKSAC.TXT

Trennert, R. A. (1998). *White man's medicine: Government doctors and the Navajo, 1863–1955.* Albuquerque: University of New Mexico Press.

Twiss, R. (2000). *One church many tribes.* Ventura, CA: Regal Books.
United States Commission on Civil Rights (USCCR). (2003). *A quiet crisis: Federal funding and unmet needs in Indian country.* Washington, DC: Author.
Weaver, H. N. (2011). Serving multicultural elders: Recommendations for helping professions. *Case Management Journal, 12*(2), 42–49. doi: 10.1891/1521-0987.12.2.42
Wilkinson, C. (2005). *Blood struggle: The rise of modern Indian nations.* New York, NY: W.W. Norton.
Zager, B. S., & Yancy, M. (2011). A call to improve practice concerning cultural sensitivity in advanced directives: A review of the literature. *Worldviews on Evidence-Based Nursing, 8*(4), 202–211. doi: 10.111/j.1741-6787.2011.00222.x
Zuckerman, S., Haley, J., Roubideaux, Y., & Lillie-Blanton, M. (2004). Health service access, use, and insurance coverage among American Indians/Alaska Natives and Whites: What role does Indian Health Services play? *American Journal of Public Health, 94*(1), 53–59.

4

Theoretical Perspectives on Aging and Physical Changes

Jane A. Tiedt

THEORIES ON AGING

Why do some people live past the century mark and others fail to make it to retirement age? Some individuals age gracefully and are full of energy and vitality well into their 80s and 90s, while others are incapacitated from diseases by the time they reach 60 years of age. Why do people age differently? Why do some people show significant cognitive decline as they age while others stay sharp and perform well in thinking skills? Why are some people debilitated from multiple losses experienced with age, yet others recover and find hope and meaning despite their losses. These questions have been pondered by researchers for decades. Despite many advances in molecular biology, biochemistry, genetics, and gerontology, these questions continue to perplex scientists. Many theories have been proposed across disciplines to explain the aging process. This chapter provides an overview of the more common biological and psychosocial theories on aging.

Biological Theories of Aging

Physically, aging begins with genetics, but as we age, biochemical and physiological processes in the body also change. Cellular and molecular biologists have proposed several theories to explain what causes aging. These are divided into two main categories. Programmed theories suggest that aging occurs based on some internal biological mechanism in our genetic code. Error theories postulate that aging is caused by prolonged environmental effects, which cause damage to our DNA, proteins, and cells. Over time, organs and body systems deteriorate and cease functioning. Before we examine these theories, a basic overview of genetics may be helpful.

The nucleus of each cell contains the genetic instructions for growth and development in the form of human DNA. Within the DNA are thousands of molecular segments or genes. One of the most important roles of genes is to direct the manufacturing of proteins such as collagen, hemoglobin, hormones, enzymes, antibodies, and antigens. The process of protein production begins when enzymes bind to the DNA. This causes the strands of the DNA to separate and a mirror image of each strand is replicated. The mirror image is called messenger RNA (mRNA). The mRNA gives instruction to the ribosomes in the cells to form a variety of amino acid polypeptides. These amino acids are released from the cell in the form of proteins. When cells get damaged or deteriorate with age, the cells simply replicate themselves through the process of mitosis. In mitosis, the chromosomes align themselves in the center of the cell. Then the DNA strands unwind and separate, and new base pairs attach to each separated section, resulting in the creation of two identical chromosomes. Then the cell divides, resulting in two cells identical to the original (Craig & Dunn, 2007).

Programmed Theories

Programmed theories assert that longevity and aging are set by our genetic code or some predetermined timetable in our genome. The premise is that an individual's life span is genetically programmed by a biological clock starting from conception. Supporters of this model are looking at the Human Genome Project to see if the aging genes can be identified. They want to see if the aging process can be slowed or postponed through pharmacogenetics (Tabloski, 2006).

In general, mammals have a relatively fixed life span. Older cells divide fewer times than younger cells. For example, fetal cells will divide about 100 times, whereas cells from an older adult stops replicating after 20 to 30 divisions (Tabloski, 2006). In humans, individuals with a more stable genetic makeup tend to live longer because they are not as vulnerable to cellular damage and mutations. Researchers believe that longevity is inherited. Children with ancestors who lived through old age are more likely to live longer than descendants of relatives who die prematurely (Davidovic et al., 2010; Jin, 2010).

Hayflick Limit

This theory was proposed in the early 1960s. Researcher Leonard Hayflick found that human cells in the laboratory environment are only capable of a finite number of divisions and then they die. With each cell division, the chromosome shortens and after 40 to 60 replications, the cell stops dividing. Our genes are specifically programmed for development and decline. This includes a set number of times a cell can reproduce through mitosis. This is known as the Hayflick limit.

Telomeres (meaning end point in Greek) are caps on the end of each chromosome. The length of the telomere is regulated by our DNA. Their role is to ensure that the chromosome strands are aligned correctly during mitosis. They also act to protect the integrity of the chromosome so that no genetic material is lost during replication. With each cell division, small amounts of the telomeres erode away. Over time, the telomeres become too short; then the chromosome can no longer divide and dies. The shortening of the telomeres contributes to aging because it limits the number of times a cell can divide. Other factors associated with shortening of the telomeres include acute and chronic stress, infection, and oxidative stress (Boyle, 2013).

Telomeres have a role in preventing broken strands of chromosomes from connecting or forming mutant strands. Telomeres are thought to have a tumor-suppressing mechanism as well. When the telomere segments shorten, genetic instability increases because there are greater chromosome breaks and translocation—where pieces of chromosomes stick together. There is no clear scientific evidence to determine the actual connection between aging and shortening telomeres (Boyle, 2013). Does this just represent a sign of aging or does the shortening telomere actually foster or accelerate aging? Some researchers hypothesize that free radicals damage the telomeres and this hastens the aging process (American Federation of Aging Research [AFAR], 2011).

Immunological

A programmed deterioration in the immune function leaves the body more susceptible to infections and diseases. This is called immunosenescence. Over time, this progressive weakening of the immune system is expressed as age-related changes and debilitating diseases. As we age, our antibodies, the body's natural defense mechanism, are less effective (Jin, 2010). As a result, we see the rates of autoimmune diseases increase with age. The immune system becomes defective and generates antibodies that attack it. This may be one factor in the development of rheumatoid arthritis, lupus, and multiple sclerosis. Some researchers posit that the aging immune system may also contribute to the development of type 2 diabetes and some types of cancers (Eiopoulos, 2010).

The programmed decrease in production of T cells (helper cells) throughout adulthood is reflected in less resistance to pathogens, and heightened susceptibility to disease. Declining effectiveness of the T cells may be manifested by increased acute infections in the elderly. This may be why we see more postoperative and hospital-acquired infections in geriatric patients. Furthermore, this population is at a greater risk for pneumonia and influenza. This makes it critical to promoting vaccinations in our senior citizens. Encouraging healthy nutritional habits high in fruits and vegetables and avoiding exposure to infectious agents can also help prevent acute infections and untimely demise.

Neuroendocrine

Our biological clock regulates hormones to control the aging process. Hormones are chemical messengers produced by the body that regulate growth, reproduction, metabolism, inflammation, stress response, and much more. The hypothalamus–pituitary–adrenal feedback loop (HPA axis) is the main pathway for regulating the hormones associated with growth and aging. The cascading actions of hormones start in the hypothalamus, which produces hormones that stimulate the pituitary. These include growth hormone-releasing factors and corticotropin-releasing hormones. The hypothalamus controls body temperature and instinctive behaviors including sex drive, thirst, hunger, and emotional reactions such as anger or aggression.

The hypothalamus and pituitary often work in conjunction with each other. Hormones released by the pituitary gland are responsible for regulating growth, maturation, and reproduction as well as controlling the adrenal cortex and thyroid. The pituitary is often called the master gland because it triggers hormones in other organs and regulates many body functions. The many hormones released by the pituitary gland include growth hormone, adrenocorticotropic hormone, thyrotropin, follicle-stimulating hormone, luteinizing hormone, antidiuretic hormone, prolactin, and oxytocin (Rathus, 2011). The pituitary is programmed to act on the gonads during puberty to stimulate the development of sex characteristics and increase production of testosterone in males and estrogen and progesterone in females. These hormones peak during early adulthood when women's bodies tend to be most fertile and in the best condition for reproduction. Menopause is biologically programmed. During middle adulthood, women's reproductive hormones decline and ovulation ends. We see physiological changes associated with declining estrogen levels including increased risk for cardiovascular disease (CVD) and osteoarthritis.

Next in the HPA feedback loop is the adrenal gland. It receives chemical messages from the hypothalamus via the pituitary gland. The adrenal gland produces corticosteroids as a part of the fight or flight response. It is responsible for regulating epinephrine and norepinephrine in the presence of actual or perceived threats and stressors (Rathus, 2011). As discussed later in this chapter, overactivation of the stress response can impair homeostasis and lead to increased risk for illness and disease. Through the relentless march of time across the decades, hormone production declines and our bodies become less responsive to their effects. As a result, researchers are focusing on the benefits of hormone replacement as a means of minimizing or reversing aging.

A visit to any nutritional supplement section at the local store demonstrates how strongly this theory is promoted in popular media. There is an overabundance of natural and synthetic hormones claiming to delay the ticking biological clock or repair the ravages of time. There is little sound scientific evidence to support these claims. In some cases, they may actually have significant risks and unwanted side effects. Supplements and hormone therapy should only be done under the supervision of a licensed health care provider (Olshansky, Hayflick, & Carnes, 2002).

Error Theories

In error theory, lifestyle and environmental factors can cause damage to DNA, RNA, and other cellular properties. The resulting damage can lead to mutations or cross-link mishaps when the DNA, mRNA, or proteins are replicated or reproduced. There is a cumulative effect from long-term damage and accumulation of mutations that impair cellular function resulting in biological decline and aging. Examples of error theories include somatic mutations, cross-link errors, damage from free radicals, and the wear-and-tear theory. Two specific examples that fall under the wear-and-tear theory include allostatic load and metabolic syndrome. In both cases, overuse of systems in the body lead to burnout and increased risk for debilitating chronic diseases.

Somatic Mutations

Constant exposure to environmental conditions and toxins can harm the DNA. Damaged DNA can usually repair itself but instability in our genes can result in greater susceptibility to mutations and errors in DNA replication. The resulting cellular or "somatic" mutations play a role in the aging process and lead to age-related diseases. Much of the knowledge about somatic mutations is based on research on the cellular damage from radiation exposure. DNA that is exposed to radiation has a shorter life span. Furthermore, as the body ages, more DNA mutations are found within the cell's mitochondria (Wong, 2001). These genetic mutations to the mitochondrial DNA cause cell malformation, deterioration, and ultimately cellular death. This can be demonstrated in chronic kidney disease, congestive heart failure, and declining immune functions commonly present in many older adults (Jin, 2010).

Cross-Link

In the cross-linked model of aging, inappropriate cross-linkages occur in DNA and protein molecules during the replication process. Over time, the damaged proteins accumulate and slow down bodily functions (Jin, 2010). The cross-linked molecules impair cellular functioning causing deficits in oxygen and nutritional uptake. This cellular damage is most noticeable in collagen. Outward signs of collagen damage include fragile, wrinkled skin and age spots. Cross-linked protein damage is hypothesized to be the cause of cataracts. Several studies in Great Britain and China are developing pharmaceuticals intended to prevent the cross-link damage that causes cataracts. Some research also suggests that the cross-link theory is linked to the development of atherosclerosis in the kidneys by impairing glucose and collagen protein binding. This results in stiffness of the renal blood vessels and declining kidney function (AFAR, 2011)

Free Radicals

Another source of cellular damage from environmental factors including pollution, smoke, alcohol, sunlight, and radiation is free radicals. The sun's ultraviolet rays create free radicals, which can damage our DNA. Free radicals are also a byproduct of cellular metabolism, chronic inflammation, and oxidative stress (Khansari, Shakiba, & Mahmoudi, 2009). We often associate oxidation with the process of rusting metal after it has been exposed to the elements. It is easy to visualize how oxidative free radicals can cause similar reactions in our bodies. Research suggests that damage in the body from free radicals increases with age (Aiken & Rudolph, 2012). Accumulation of free radicals is theorized to contribute to the development of cancers, CVD, diabetes, arthritis, and atherosclerosis (AFAR, 2011).

A free radical is a molecule that has a free electron, which makes it highly reactive. These free radicals attach to other molecules by adding oxygen. Mitochondria in the cells metabolize 90% of the body's oxygen, so they are extremely vulnerable to oxidative stress (Khansari et al., 2009). When mitochondria generate energy for the cell, oxygen free radicals are one of the by-products. Furthermore, with repeated exposure to free radicals, this metabolic process becomes impaired. As the damage to the mitochondria increases, they produce less energy and generate more free radicals. It becomes a vicious cycle leading to cellular destruction. Further damage occurs when the free radicals attach to protein molecules. The protein's behavior change results in cellular, tissue, and organ dysfunction.

Antioxidants have been shown to be beneficial in reducing and repairing damage caused by free radicals. Naturally occurring antioxidants include vitamins A, B_6, B_{12}, C, E, folic acid, beta-carotene, and selenium. Consuming diets high in fruits and vegetables can help reduce the risk of oxidative stress–related diseases. On the other hand, there is little scientific evidence to support the antiaging benefits of taking antioxidant supplements (Cui, Jing, & Pan, 2013c; Jiang et al., 2010; Rosenbaum, O'Mathuna, Chavez, & Shields, 2010).

Wear and Tear

Aging results from progressive damage to cells and tissues. The premise of the wear-and-tear theory is that cells, tissue, and organs wear out with repeated action and misuse. As cells, they are replaced with new ones. With age, the body has a diminished capacity to repair itself. Recurring injuries can also lead to permanent disability. This theory can be demonstrated in the professional baseball pitcher who has thrown millions of pitches throughout his career and experiences chronic joint pain from years of overuse. Other examples are carpal tunnel syndrome or tennis elbow. Both result from chronic repetitive movements that cause wear and tear to joints, cartilage, and tissue. Like a machine, the human body wears out from constant use and abuse. For example, the cells that line artery walls deteriorate faster in the presence of chronic hypertension. Protective measures and good health habits can decrease wear and tear and prolong vitality and longevity (Jin, 2010; Wong, 2001).

Allostatic Load

Constant worries and daily pressures cause certain biochemical reactions in our body in order to produce energy to cope with the stressor. Hormones are released that cause the heart rate and blood pressure to increase and mobilize energy stores. Allostasis is the adaptive process of maintaining balance in the body during the stress response (McEwen & Laskey, 2003). It involves the production of adrenaline, cortisol, and other chemical messengers through the activation of neurochemical pathways. Chronic repetitive activation of this system results in allostatic load.

McEwen (2005) introduced this term to explain the wear and tear on the body and brain caused by chronic activation of the stress response. This mechanism becomes less efficient over time or simply is overwhelmed by too many stressors. The process is detrimental if the strain persists and the stress response continues as a heightened state of arousal. It can lead to a weakened immune system; increase risks of stomach ulcers, fatigue, depression, osteoporosis, CVD, and type 2 diabetes; as well as accelerate the aging process (Ropeik, 2004; Sapolsky, 2004). Allostatic load is not a malfunction of the system, but results from chronic overuse. Allostatic load is considered one of the links between stress and disease.

Metabolic Syndrome

As early as the 1960s, scientists were noticing a relationship between CVD, triglyceride levels, and diabetes (Ginsberg, 1993). About 20 years ago, the term metabolic syndrome or syndrome X was coined for a cluster of clinical factors associated with increased risk for diabetes and CVD. These include dyslipidemia, hypertension, impaired glucose metabolism, hyperinsulinemia, and impaired prothrombolytic and proinflammatory states. According to the Adult Treatment Panel III study issued by the National Cholesterol Education Program, the presence of three or more of these risk factors is diagnostic for metabolic syndrome (Weir & Lipscombe, 2004). In an analysis of data from the third National Health and Nutrition Examination Survey (NHANES) study, 44% of Americans older than 50 years had metabolic syndrome (Ford, Giles, & Dietz, 2002).

If left untreated, metabolic syndrome causes chronic inflammation. It appears to accelerate aging and is associated with decreased life expectancy and increased morbidity.

Several studies have delved into the link between obesity, insulin resistance, hypertension, hyperlipidemia, CVD, and diabetes. They have begun to look at the molecular pathways among obesity, diabetes, and the inflammatory marker tumor necrosis factor-alpha (TNF-α). This inflammatory marker is overproduced in the fat cells of obese mice and is also present in the muscle cells of obese humans. After injecting TNF-α into obese mice, their insulin function became impaired. The researchers concluded that TNF-α inhibits insulin receptor signaling pathways (IRS-1). This IRS-1 pathway is the key mechanism by which stress and inflammation lead to insulin resistance (Wellen & Hotamisligil, 2005). Elevated insulin and glucose levels increase oxidative stress and the production of free radicals. In turn, oxygen free radicals impair insulin-sensitive glucose transporters on the cell membrane and insulin resistance results (Banks & Morley, 2000).

PSYCHOSOCIAL THEORIES

Life Course Theory

When looking at psychosocial theories of aging, it is important to consider historical, cultural, social, economic, and political contexts. Cohorts, or those individuals born during the same time period, are connected by life events. People born during the Great Depression, after World War II (WWII), or in the new millennium are all examples of different cohort groups. Over the course of a lifetime, each cohort develops unique characteristics as these historic events shape their beliefs, values, habits, and ways of life. This life course model looks at cohorts as they are situated in place and time. This means that age norms, roles, and role transitions such as habits, gender roles, and expected behavior during retirement are similar within a cohort group. Life course elements may include income, education, neighborhood, social institutions, and political and world events. These can have positive or negative effects on aging, well-being, and physical condition over the life span (Hertzman, 2004).

Continuity Theory

In the continuity theory, aging is just viewed as a normal part of life, and habits and idiosyncrasies persist from childhood through adulthood. The continuation of these traits carries over into preferences for roles and social interactions (Atchley, 1989). Enduring personality traits such as dependence, moodiness, outgoing, sensitivity, and confidence can all influence a person's adaptability to aging. Some older people will feel a loss of identity or self-esteem after retiring, while others develop a new positive sense of self. They substitute new roles for old ones as a means of adjusting to their changing environment. Some seek change while others mourn the loss of identity. For many, there is a balance between positive traits, which offset the negative effects associated with aging (Aiken & Rudolph, 2012).

Disengagement Theory

The disengagement theory proposed by Cummings and Henry more than 50 years ago focuses on loss and isolation associated with aging. The underlying premise of the theory is there is a joint withdrawal process between society and the elderly that helps maintain societal equilibrium. The disengagement theory was linked to post-WWII-era retiring seniors. They were freed from previous roles and job obligations to make way for the next generation of workers. This release from responsibilities occurs in conjunction with declining physical and mental capacities (Atchley, 1989). Retirement is a voluntary act of disentanglement, allowing retirees a chance to slow down and gradually withdraw from social events and social circles. This frees up time for more reflection and reminiscence. Disengagement provides faulty justification for isolating the elderly based on the presumption that it is what they desire, when in reality many older adults prefer to remain actively involved with society (Howe, 1987).

Activity Theory

Robert Havighurst proposed this theory to refute notions presented in the disengagement theory. The activity theory from the field of sociology suggests that there is a positive relationship among life satisfaction, social interactions, and activity levels in the elderly. This theory is really an antiaging approach to living out the senior years. It embraces the notion of use it or lose it as the basis for healthy aging. The goal of activity theory is to suspend functional decline associated with aging and delay the onset of disease and demise (Aiken & Rudolph, 2012). Research supports the premise that age-associated decline can be postponed or prevented by engaging in long-term physical activity (Fries, 2012). Older adults are happier when they are physically and cognitively engaged. Quality of life is enhanced when older people pursue activities that give them pleasure.

As roles change with age, it is important to find substitute roles and activities in order to stay engaged. A longitudinal study of 538 participants from a 50-plus runners club compared them to 423 age-matched controls, and followed them over the next 30 years. The researcher found that the disability differences grew significantly between the groups as they aged. The runner group had lower levels of disability, which did not increase as fast or as much as the control group (Fries, 2012). Being active throughout the life span reduces age-related deterioration. A study by Booth and Zwetsloot (2010) found that 80-year-old senior citizens who were physically active throughout their life had similar muscle strength and aerobic capacity as sedentary individuals who were 50 to 55 years of age. The results support the underlying premise of the activity theory.

Erikson's Stage of Integrity Versus Despair

Some behavioral scientists have proposed developmental tasks associated with aging. Successful attainment of these tasks leads to pleasure, fulfillment, and the ability to perform and succeed in subsequent developmental tasks. Failure leads to unhappiness, disappointment, and difficulty in attaining later tasks. Erik Erikson was a neo-Freudian. His theory is derived from Freud's psychosexual stages, but Erikson recognized that there are also many social aspects that influence human development. Erikson's psychosocial theory emphasizes how social systems influence the development of personality. He proposed that individuals move through eight stages over the life span (Erikson, Erikson, & Kivnick, 1986). During each stage, a person must resolve a particular conflict before moving on to the next stage. Erikson's final stage is integrity versus despair. Adults, aged 65 years and older, are confronted with the issue of, "Has my life been meaningful?" When contemplating life accomplishments, many seniors ask the question, "If I had to live my life over, what would I do differently?" If they feel that there is little they would change then they have achieved a healthy sense of integrity. If they view life as a series of failures and have a lot of regrets and unresolved conflict, then they may feel a sense of despair (Sigelman & Rider, 2006).

As seniors look back in their old age, are they satisfied because their life had meaning and purpose? Did they live up to their dreams and expectations? Did they do the best they could despite the circumstances? All of these positive perspectives will lead to the development of integrity. Instead, does their life seem full of missed opportunities, wrong choices, unmet needs, or strained relations? These may lead to feelings of despair and hopelessness. The life review process allows elders to reminisce and come to terms with disappointments, find meaning, and prepare for death with peace of mind rather than regrets. Satisfactory attainment of this stage is a balance between realizing that not everything turns out as planned, but also recognizing that life has had positive rewards and those outweigh the regrets (Erikson & Erikson, 1997).

Peck's Stages of Older Adulthood

Robert Peck expanded on Erikson's theory by dividing the integrity stage into three tasks of old age based on the psychosocial and physical losses experienced in old age. He suggested that aging could be an opportunity for change by being flexible and staying positive. The first task for aging is ego differentiation versus work-role preoccupation. Before retirement, people define themselves in terms of family life and occupation. They can become preoccupied with their work role. Life events such as retirement, divorce, or adult children leaving home create a void in their identity. The task of this stage is for older adults to redefine themselves. Retirees can do this by recognizing the gifts of expertise they have developed from well-established careers. They should look for ways to mentor the next generation rather than becoming focused on loss of status or prestige they had gained throughout their career. They need to find satisfaction in retirement and seeing their adult children launching their own careers. According to Peck's model, in this first stage, older adults need to change how they identify themselves and look for opportunities to redefine their roles: grandparent, mentor, volunteer, even student. Embrace the period as a time to learn new things.

The second phase of old age in Peck's model is body transcendence versus body preoccupation. As we age, many noticeable physical changes occur. Organ reserves decline. Even the most physically active seniors require longer recovery times after exercise as they age. Aging immune systems are less able to ward off infection and disease. Outward physical manifestations of aging are visibly apparent, but seniors should not become self-absorbed with these physical changes. The goal is to avoid dwelling on limitations and ailments associated with aging otherwise seniors become sullen and depressed. Rather, seniors have acquired a lifetime of knowledge and wisdom to share and must focus more on these positives. The goal of this stage is for seniors to develop skills to see beyond daily aches and pains or a declining physical body, and look for ways to have a meaningful life despite the physical deterioration and illness concerns. Seniors should appreciate what cognitive skills and social connections that are still in place, and learn to accept things and enjoy the good days. They should recognize that there are always options, and should choose to live in gratitude.

Ego transcendence versus ego preoccupation is Peck's final stage of late adulthood. The elderly can ruminate over the many losses experienced and their own impending mortality. Or, they can choose to recognize what they have contributed to the world even in small ways and how these life contributions will live on when they are gone. The elderly should avoid becoming obsessed with death and dying. Shift their focus to the joy of being connected to the next generation and reflecting on life rather than dwelling on the limited future. Encourage them to look at how they can leave a legacy by sharing their knowledge, wisdom, and gifts with future generations (Craig & Dunn, 2007).

SUMMARY

Most scientists agree that development and aging are both products of nature and nurture. Although our genetics may set the stage for the aging process, exposure to environmental forces over a lifetime can have acute and long-term consequences. As these theories suggest, aging involves biological, psychological, and social dimensions. Societal and cultural values and norms, learning, and experiences can have profound effects. Changes can occur suddenly or slowly. People gradually gain wrinkles, lose visual acuity, or can suddenly lose speech or body functions after a stroke or brain aneurysm. Nursing's role is to help elderly clients adjust to the changes, both positive and negative, that are associated with aging. It is our responsibility to optimize their health in order to promote quality of life and minimize disability. Nurses can encourage participation in activities that support the client's interests and skills while respecting a client's needs for autonomy and decision making. It is our role to maximize these opportunities.

RESOURCES

Merck Manual

www.merckmanuals.com/home/older_peoples_health_issues/the_aging_body/changes_in_the_body_with_aginger.html

Search Terms
- Overview of aging
- Disorders in older people
- Changes in the body
- Accelerated aging

National Institute of Health

www.nlm.nih.gov/medlineplus/ency/article/004012.htm

Search Terms
- Aging changes in organs tissues and cells
- Aging theory
- Common terms

REFERENCES

Aiken, M., & Rudolph, M. (2012). Biological and social theories of aging. In R. Padilla, S. Byers-Cannon, & H. Lohman (Eds.), *OT for elders* (3rd ed., pp. 21–30). St. Louis, MO: Mosby.

American Federation of Aging Research (AFAR). (2011). *Theories of aging.* New York, NY: Author. Retrieved from www.AFAR.org/docs/migrated/11121_infoaging_guide_theories_of_aging_FG.pdf

Atchley, R. C. (1989). A continuity theory of normal aging. *The Gerontologist, 29*(2), 183–190. doi: 10.1093/geront/29.2.183

Banks, W. A., & Morley, J. E. (2000). Endocrine and metabolic changes in human aging. *Journal of the American Aging Association, 23*(2), 103–115.

Booth, F. W., & Zwetsloot, K. A. (2010). Basic concepts about genes, inactivity and aging. *Scandinavian Journal of Medicine and Science in Sports, 20*(1), 1–4. doi: 10.1111/j.1600-0838.2009.00972x

Boyle, M. M. (2013). Telomeres, cancer and aging. *Journal of the Australian Traditional-Medicine Society, 19*(3), 154–159.

Craig, G. J., & Dunn, W. L. (2007). *Understanding human development.* Upper Saddle River, NJ: Pearson Education.

Cui, Y. H., Jing, C. X., & Pan, H. W. (2013). Association of blood antioxidants and vitamins with risk of age-related cataract: A meta-analysis of observational studies. *American Journal of Clinical Nutrition, 98*(3), 778–786. doi: 10.3945/ajcn.112.053835

Davidovic, M., Sevo, G., Svorcan, P., Milosevic, D. P., Despotovic, N., & Erceg, P. (2010). Old age as a privilege of the "selfish ones." *Aging and Disease, 1*(2), 139–146.

Eiopoulos, C. (2010). *Gerontological nursing* (7th ed.). Philadelphia, PA: Lippincott, Williams & Wilkins.

Erikson, E. H., & Erikson, J. W. (1997). *The life cycle completed.* New York, NY: Norton.

Erikson, E. H., Erikson, J. W., & Kivnick, H. (1986). *Vital involvement in old age.* New York, NY: Norton.

Ford, E. S., Giles, W. H., & Dietz, W. H. (2002). Prevalence of the metabolic syndrome among US adults: Findings from the third National Health and Nutrition Examination Survey. *JAMA: The Journal of the American Medical Association, 287*(3), 356–359. doi: 10.1001/jama.287.3.356

Fries, J. F. (2012). The theory and practice of active aging. *Current Gerontology and Geriatrics Research, 2012,* 420637.

Ginsberg, H. N. (1993). Syndrome X: what's old, what's new, what's etiologic? *The Journal of Clinical Investigation, 92*(1), 3.

Hertzman, C. (2004). The life-course contribution to ethnic disparities in health. In N. B. Anderson, R. A. Bulatao, & B. Cohen (Eds.), *Critical perspectives on racial and ethnic differences in health in later life* (pp. 143–170). Washington, DC: National Academies Press. Retrieved from http://www.nap.edu/openbook.php?record_id=11086&page=143

Howe, C. Z. (1987). Selected social gerontology theories and older adult leisure involvement: A review of the literature. *Journal of Applied Gerontology, 6*, 448–463. doi: 10.1077/073346488700600407

Jiang, L., Yang, K., Tian, J., Guan, Q., Yao, N., Cao, N., … Yang, S. (2010). Efficacy of antioxidant vitamins and selenium supplement in prostate cancer prevention: A meta-analysis of randomized control trials. *Nutrition and Cancer, 62*(6), 719–727. doi: 10.1080/01635581.2010.494335

Jin, K. (2010). Modern biological theories of aging. *Aging and Disease, 1*(2), 72–74.

Khansari, N., Shakiba, Y., & Mahmoudi, M. (2009). Chronic inflammation and oxidative stress as a major cause of age-related diseases and cancer. *Recent Patents on Inflammation & Allergy Drug Discovery, 3*(1), 73–80. doi: 10.2174/187221309787158371

McEwen, B. S. (2005). Stressed or stressed out: What is the difference? *Journal of Psychiatry & Neuroscience, 30*(5), 315–318.

McEwen, B., & Lasley, E. N. (2003). Allostatic load: When protection gives way to damage. *Advances in Mind-Body Medicine, 19*(1), 28–33.

Olshansky, S. J., Hayflick, L., & Carnes, B. A. (2002). Position statement on human aging. *The Journals of Gerontology, 57*(8), B292–B297. doi: 10.1013/Geront/57.8.B292

Rathus, S. (2011). *Psychology: Concepts and connections* (10th ed). Belmont, CA: Wadsworth Cengage Learning.

Ropeik, D. (2004). The consequence of fear. *EMBO Reports, 5*(S1), S56–S60.

Rosenbaum, C. C., O'Mathuna, D. P., Chavez, M., & Shields, K. (2010). Antioxidants and anti-inflammatory dietary supplements for osteoarthritis and rheumatoid arthritis. *Alternative Therapies in Health and Medicine. 16*(2), 32–40. Retrieved from http://www.encognitive.com/files/antioxidants%20and%20antiinflammatory%20dietary%20supplements%20for%20osteoarthritis%20and%20rheumatoid%20arthritis.pdf

Sapolsky, R. (2004). *Why zebras don't get ulcers* (3rd ed.). New York, NY: Owl Books.

Sigelman, C. K., & Rider, E. A. (2006). *Life-span human development* (5th ed.). Belmont, CA: Thomson Higher Education.

Tabloski, P. A. (2006). *Gerontological nursing.* Upper Saddle River, NJ: Pearson-Prentice Hall.

Weir, E., & Lipscombe, L. (2004). Metabolic syndrome: Waist not, want not. *Canadian Medical Association Journal, 170*(9), 1390–1391.

Wellen, K. E., & Hotasmisligil, G. S. (2005). Inflammation, stress, and diabetes. *Journal of Clinical Investigations, 115*(5), 1111–1120.

Wong, T. P. (2001). An old question revisited: Current understanding of aging theories. *McGill Journal of Medicine, 6*(1), 41–47.

5

How to Deal With Compromised Independence

Brenda L. Bonham Howe

PHYSICAL AND MENTAL CHANGES OF AGING

Aging is a normal part of the human life span. However, in the past century, many Americans experienced life-extending benefits of modern medicine. Increased mobility, marketing, and refrigeration improved the variety of fresh foods available year round for a large part of the population. The Industrial Revolution brought about changes in work patterns, which allowed more individuals an opportunity for relaxation and recreation. Public health and sanitation improvements decreased the spread of disease (Dewald, 2014). The 20th century brought advances in science and medication that resulted in better health education, prevention and treatment of disease, and, thus, longer lives for a significant portion of the world's population. However, science still has its limits and the inevitable happens as our bodies do not regenerate.

PHYSICAL CHANGES ASSOCIATED WITH AGING

Vision

Visual changes occur with aging without precipitating disease factors. Individuals who have never needed visual aids (glasses or contacts) will find a need for reading glasses sometime in their 40s as the eye lenses become less flexible (presbyopia). As years pass, night vision decreases and glare interferes with vision. Driving in the dark when it is raining increases the risk of accidents for many people (WebMD, 2012).

Vision also plays a role in safe mobility. The ability to see where one is going and changes in terrain and texture are all important aspects of walking. The risk of injuries increases with the visual changes that come with normal aging or as a result of disease processes (diabetes, glaucoma, cataracts, detached retina, cancer, shingles).

It is important to remember that some medications may also interfere with vision. Educating clients and caregivers about potential side effects of new medications or increased doses is important. Remind them to always report side effects to their health care provider right away.

The loss of vision can contribute to loss of independence, inability to participate in favorite pastime activities, injury, loss of socialization, and depression.

Vision Loss Interventions

Many potential changes may occur with vision after the age of 40 years. The American Ophthalmology Association (AOA) recommends an annual medication review and visual acuity examination (AOA, 2014). It is also important to keep eyeglasses clean and in good repair as this helps to keep them in appropriate alignment with the wearer's visual field, reducing visual distortion.

Multiple circumstances contribute to the inability of many people to follow through with annual eye examinations. It is the health care professional's role to educate individuals about the importance of recommended examinations. Early diagnosis increases the likelihood of postponing additional decline in visual health status.

Hearing Problems

According to Dr. Li-Korotky (2012), "age-related hearing loss is the third most prevalent chronic condition in older Americans after hypertension and arthritis, and is a leading cause of adult hearing handicaps in the United States." Hearing loss may begin early in life due to frequent exposure to noise. Damage to the hearing apparatus may occur gradually over a long period of time. Acute hearing loss may result after an accident, illness, or proximity to explosions associated with construction or war. Age-related hearing loss (ARHL) affects millions of geriatric individuals.

Any form of hearing loss reduces environmental stimulations, which may diminish pleasure associated with birds singing, pets making noises, music, and favorite television or radio programs. Communicating by phone may be compromised, which can contribute to a feeling of social isolation. Quality person-to-person communication becomes impaired as tone nuances are lost. The inability to hear can frustrate the individual, contributing to irritability. Caregivers who must raise their voices may also experience frustration as trying to communicate this way can be a physical and emotional drain.

Research indicates that ARHL may aggravate cognitive decline. Cognitive impairment may contribute to poor speech and understanding. These factors associated with multisensory mechanisms may contribute to difficulty coping with everyday settings (Li-Korotky, 2012).

Hearing Loss Intervention

As with all potential health problems, early detection is key. A medication review should be the first step of assessment in the event that hearing changes represent adverse side effects.

Early prevention includes having an awareness of constant background noises, which may contribute to hearing loss. Wearing protective auditory devices, when appropriate, will help to reduce long-term nerve damage.

Family members complain about the volume of the television, "He cranks that volume to the top and it gives me a headache. But he can't hear it if the volume is lower and he refuses to be checked for hearing aids." Or, "We got grandma a headset for the TV, but she won't use it." Loud noises can fray the nerves and potentially trigger aggressive behavior in the elderly (especially with dementia present). When an elderly adult lives with a family member(s), the loud TV may contribute to frustration. If the problem is not resolved in some mutually agreeable manner, it may become a constant source of conflict.

It may be helpful to approach the elder to explain that the loud noise can cause hearing impairment for the other family members. The resistance to a hearing examination may be due to embarrassment or fear. Explain that hearing tests are much improved as are hearing assistive devices.

The potential to regain some hearing ability would improve quality of life for the hearing impaired and for those living in the same household.

When a hearing-impaired person moves into an assisted living or skilled care community, there may be rules about media volume. If that is the case, then assistive hearing devices may become necessary.

MUSCULOSKELETAL CHANGES

Dr. LeBrasseur (2014) states, "We achieve peak muscle mass by our early 40s, and have a progressive deterioration from that point on, resulting in as much as a 50 percent loss by the time we are in our 80s or 90s" (Mayo Clinic, 2014). Loss of muscle strength and skeletal changes lead to mobility challenges. Mobility impediments contribute to falls and the additional risk of broken bones, damaged nerves, and increased anxiety. Loss of muscle mass and strength also results in less flexibility and physical energy. Some of the most frequently diagnosed musculoskeletal disorders include fractures, osteoporosis, osteoarthritis, microcrystal disorders, infections, and tumors (Gheno, Cepparo, Rosca, & Cotton, 2012). Many of these disorders contribute to acute and chronic pain, which often require some level of medication management.

Fatigue is a common complaint of the geriatric generation, but is not always due to musculoskeletal changes. Medications that may contribute to fatigue include antianxiety medicines, antidepressants, blood pressure medicines, and statins for high cholesterol (WebMD, 2013). Comorbidities such as congestive heart failure and arthritis reduce energy levels (National Institute on Aging/National Institutes of Health [NIA/NIH], 2014).

All of these concerns contribute to falls, which can instantly change the life of that individual. One out of three adults older than 65 years falls each year. The Centers for Disease Control and Prevention (CDC) stated in 2010 that 2.3 million nonfatal fall injuries occurred among older adults who were assessed by a health care provider (many falls go unreported). The same year more than 662,000 patients were hospitalized due to falls. This information does not reflect how many minor injuries occurred due to elder falls, nor does it clarify the number of fractures that occurred in the spine, hip, forearm, leg, ankle, pelvis, upper arm, and hand (CDC, 2014). The fear of falling may also contribute to less activity, further deconditioning, and exacerbation of poor health.

Musculoskeletal Interventions

Rehabilitation may provide individuals with improved muscle strength. With better metabolic function every system benefits: better circulation, improved oxygenation, mental function, and hope for some restoration of independence. Early intervention is ideal, but too often it comes about due to a fall or other health problem that presses elders to seek medical advice (Central Vermont Medical Center [CVMC], 2014).

Surgical intervention may also be a necessary form of treatment in order to restore mobility. The National Hospital Discharge Survey showed that 719,000 total knee replacements and 332,000 total hip replacement surgeries were performed in 2010 (CDC, 2010).

It is always important to conduct a review of medications to identify if any of them contributes to unwanted symptoms (Ziere et al., 2006). Education of clients and caregivers may improve understanding of the importance of regular exercise (even chair exercises), will prevent further loss of strength, and may even improve strength. Assisting the client in making community connections, such as an exercise program at a senior center, may lead to positive improvement and quality of life. If the individual is not able to leave home, it is possible for a health care provider to order an assessment in the home by a home health physical therapist.

FOOT HEALTH

Most people take better care of the tires on their car than their feet, yet feet are the primary source of mobility for a greater portion of the population. Fashion often dictates the type of shoes selected instead of shoes that fit well and that provide proper support and comfort. Shoes that do not fit well contribute to several common foot problems: corns, calluses, fissures, plantar fasciitis, achilles tendonitis, bunions, and painful neuromas (American Podiatric Medical Association [APMA], 2014). Years of wearing inadequate footwear also contribute to age-related deterioration of the balance and neuromuscular systems (Menant et al., 2008). Diseases such as arthritis, diabetes, and cardiovascular disease greatly increase the risk for neuralgia, infection, and amputation.

Onychomycosis (toenail fungus) is a very common geriatric foot problem. A fungus is an opportunistic microorganism that lives on the human body. When a break in the protective layer of skin occurs, fungi will follow. Skin, nail, and hair changes that occur with aging include loss of collagen, an incomplete protein that strengthens the tissue and contributes to dryness of skin and brittleness of nails. The nails become microscopically porous. The porous, warm, dark, and moist environment with nutrients is enough for fungi to move in and grow. Many people have multiple fungal affected nails that contribute to the following:

- Thick, opaque nails, which are very difficult to trim
- Toe of shoe presses against thick fungal nails causing tenderness, inflammation, and pressure wounds on the nail bed
- Thick, irregular overgrowth of nails press into other toes, causing skin breakdown and infection
- The unsightly nature of fungal nails causes embarrassment and hesitation to ask others to trim the nails
- Common tendency is to hide the nails from sight, keeping the feet and toes in a dark, moist, and warm environment
- People sometimes buy shoes a size larger to accommodate the thickness or the extra length of their nails if they cannot see, reach, or manipulate clippers, which may increase the risk of trips and falls

Footwear has been identified as an environmental risk factor for indoor and outdoor falls (Menant et al., 2008). When combined with any of the common foot disorders, the possibility of a fall increases. One shoe style that contributes to falls is slippers or moccasins. These are soft, accommodate tired, sore feet and deformities, and require no bending over to lace or fasten.

Menant et al. (2008) obtained a sample of 312 older community-dwelling people: those who wore slippers indoors versus no shoes or fastened shoes reported more foot pain, and had a significantly greater fall risk score as indicated by deficits in sensorimotor function tests (visual contrast sensitivity, knee extension strength, proprioception, postural sway, and hand reaction time; Menant et al., 2008).

Foot Health Intervention

A professional foot assessment (see the Appendix to this chapter) is the best place to start. Anyone may access a foot assessment form from the Lower Extremity Amputation Prevention (LEAP) website (see Resources at the end of the chapter) to understand how many particulars of the feet are included in a medical assessment. It is possible to locate a foot care nurse by checking local home health agencies, senior centers, or seniors and persons with disabilities. The American Foot Care Association (AFCA) website has a search link to locate members across the United States. Primary health care providers are qualified to perform lower limb and foot care assessment. The assessment may take 15 minutes, so it is important to schedule the time.

The most in-depth assessment of feet needs to be made by a podiatrist. According to the APMA (2014), "A podiatrist is a doctor of podiatric medicine (DPM), also known as a podiatric physician or surgeon. Podiatrists diagnose and treat conditions of the foot, ankle, and related structures of the leg." Podiatrists assess the lower legs, ankles, feet, and also evaluate balance and gait cycle. Abnormalities in gait and balance affect the whole musculoskeletal system. Irregularities of gait cause wear and tear on the ankles, strain on the knees and hips, and precipitate low back pain. The feet are the foundation of the skeletal structure. When the foundation is unsteady, the structure is stressed. Sometimes an excellent shoe fit can improve all symptoms that originated from foot neglect due to knowledge deficit, style preference, finances, or lack of access.

Shoe styles to avoid are those with soft soles, elevated heel heights, rocker-bottom sole designs, shoes that are too narrow or too wide, or are uncomfortable at the start. Those that are made with a wider sole and a superior collar of upper materials are desirable. No shoe should need to be "broken in." If the shoe is not comfortable at the store, do not take the pair home.

Shoe choices that can assist an older individual with balance are: (a) avoiding shoes with elevated heel heights (unless the patient has a severe ankle dorsiflexion limitation of the ankle joint), excessively soft sole material, or rocker-bottom sole designs; and (b) selecting shoes with wider sole material and a more superior collar of the upper materials. Going about with bare feet is not advisable for older adults or for anyone with neuropathy. Loss of fat padding from the bottom of the feet contributes to foot pain (for those who still feel their feet), the potential for picking up foreign objects (needles, tacks), or experiencing trauma (Gross, 2010). Walking barefoot also contributes to friction-induced dry skin and callus formation on the soles of the feet.

Diagnosis and treatment of common conditions (corns, calluses, fissures, etc.) may only require protection or padding with thin sponge, moleskin, or toe sleeves. Thin ribbons of medical lambs' wool are often used to weave between toes to provide wicking of moisture and to prevent skin breakdown. A variety of topical treatments may be recommended for treatment of fungal toenails. Although these treatments may seem simple, the key to success with them is consistent use and that is sometimes a challenge.

Routine nail care is important, especially for all older adults, because the nails have the potential of causing pain, altering gait, and providing access to infection. It is unfortunate that Medicare only pays for podiatrist or primary care provider delivery of foot and nail care every 60 days. This service is limited to individuals with diabetes or severe circulatory impairment to the feet. It is unfortunate that thousands of middle-aged and older citizens who can no longer see or reach their toenails (and who perhaps cannot maneuver clippers) are financially responsible for professional foot and nail care. This becomes a great obstacle for many who subsist on a limited income (see Resources at the end of the chapter).

MEMORY LOSS AND AGING

Age-related memory loss is a normal part of the aging process. Forgetting someone's name temporarily or the inability to think of a certain word is an example of normal age-related memory loss. Many times the word or name is recalled later in the day, and often without trying to remember it. This type of memory challenge does not prevent an individual from living a full and active life. It is still possible to live and work independently, maintain friendships, and even take care of others.

There are several potential diagnoses for memory loss, and memory loss may also be staged in several levels according to symptoms. The purpose of this section is not to identify the various causes, but to discuss memory loss and the challenges it presents to the individual and family members or caregivers.

The most common symptoms of memory loss include diminished:

- Ability to learn
- Thinking and making sound judgments
- Mathematical skills
- Initiative
- Attention span

Potential changes include:

- Personality: Outgoing person withdraws, a kind person becomes uncaring
- Emotions are not well controlled; agitation, depression, and suspiciousness may develop

Many people report that the most difficult symptoms are:

- Inability to communicate
- Inability to recognize family and close friends

- Loss of independence, including driving
- Being aware of memory changes
- Inability to perform daily tasks
- Repetition of phrases or stories
- Wandering
- Loss of social inhibition (public displays of sexuality)
- Accusations of stealing
- Profanity, often not part of the person's vocabulary prior to memory changes
- Unable to rationalize current condition with potential safety risks

Memory Loss Interventions

As with all health concerns, early diagnosis improves the potential for treatment with quality outcomes. A review of medications is important, followed by a discussion of advances in treating memory loss. Age-related memory loss usually occurs slowly and many of us use notes to prompt our memory regarding phone numbers, names, ideas, appointments, one's address, and directions to one's home. Other techniques to offset memory loss include:

- Adhere sticky notes around the house with reminders such as "Check door locks before bedtime," "Order B/P med on Tues"
- Label cupboards and drawers with words or pictures that describe their contents
- Keep key phone numbers next to the phone
- Schedule reminder phone calls from family, friends, or services: time for pills, time for lunch, and so on
- Use a wall calendar to keep track of time and to remember important dates
- Label photos with names and relationships (daughter, friend) and place in sight or on a bulletin board
- Keep track of phone messages by using an answering machine

- Use a spiral binder to make daily notes, "Took my pills at 8 a.m. with breakfast," "Replaced hearing aid batteries," and so on
- Use a white erase board, placed in a high-traffic area, for ongoing or daily reminders ("Today is Mon, June 4" or "Appt. with Dr. Jones on Friday, June 7 at 10 a.m. for lab results"; Saczynski & Rebok, 2004)

ALZHEIMER'S DISEASE

Alzheimer's disease progresses through stages of "early," "middle," and "late." Symptoms increase at each stage; therefore, the care and oversight needed are adjusted as the need arises. It is helpful for all involved to understand what lies ahead in order to cope as well as possible. The Alzheimer's Organization offers extensive information at www.alz.org under the headings of: What is Alzheimer's?, Caregiving, 10 Warning Signs, Seven Stages, and Search by State.

Many family members try to keep their memory-impaired loved one at home as long as possible. Making slight changes in the environment can improve some of the safety risks. Accidents happen even in safe environments, so having a first-aid kit is advisable. Small changes made over time are less likely to add to the confusion and may help avoid agitation. Changes may be needed to simplify life; remove clutter and even put artificial fruit out of sight (if it looks real, eating it may be attempted). Bottles of aftershave, lotion, shampoo, detergent, and chemicals may all be seen as something to drink. Keep keys, eyeglasses, wallet, and purse in a location where they will not be picked up by the afflicted and placed somewhere they cannot be found easily.

Caregivers

Providing 24/7 care for someone with significant memory loss can be an exhausting and emotionally draining experience. Caregivers often put aside their own needs in order to take care of a loved one.

It is not unusual for caregivers to suffer health issues to the point of collapsing under the strain (McDaniel, 2012). Caregivers may be encouraged to seek additional support through a variety of community services. Chapters in this book provide information about a variety of volunteer and in-home services that may alleviate some of the caregiver stress. As symptoms increase, caregiver fatigue sets in and it may be time to consider the option of a memory care facility where 24/7 supervision is provided. There is a growing need for memory care facilities and new ones are planned and being implemented across the United States. It is a growing specialty area with new insights and strategies to improve the quality of life for these individuals. Facilities always have someone available to discuss arrangements and potential payment sources.

SUMMARY

- There are several causes of loss of independence.
- Physical changes include loss of vision, hearing, and mobility (standing, walking, reaching, and lifting).
- Cognitive changes may be due to aging or disease processes.
- Safety for the afflicted and the caregiver can become a concern.
- Resources for how to maintain quality of life are provided.

RESOURCES

Alzhelmer's Organization

http://www.alz.org

Search Terms
- What is Alzheimer's?
- Caregiving
- Seven stages
- 10 warning signs

American Foot Care Nurse Association

www.afcna.org

Search Terms
- What is a foot care nurse?
- Find a foot care nurse in your area
- Charity care—pay it forward
- Foot care newsletters
- Foot care resources and videos

American Optometric Association

http://www.aoa.org/patients-and-public/eye-and-vision-problems

Search Terms
- Case manager cataract
- Glaucoma
- Diabetic retinopathy

Case Management Society of America

http://www.cmsa.org

Search Terms
- Consumer, discover how a case manager can help you

Exercise and Mobility

Caring-for-Aging-Parents.com
http://www.caring-for-aging-parents.com/exercises-for-the-elderly.html

Search Terms
- Exercises for the elderly
- Physical benefits

- Mental benefits
- Examples of exercise

Lower Extremity Amputation Prevention (LEAP)

http://www.hrsa.gov/hansensdisease/leap

Search Terms
- Five-Step LEAP Program
- Level-three foot inspection
- Patient education
- Footwear

Medical Alert Systems

http://www.consumersadvocate.org/medical-alerts/best-medical-alerts?utm_source=Bing&utm_medium=PaidSearch&utm_campaign=MedicalAlerts&utm_term=medical%20alert%20systems%20comparison

Search Terms
- Contract
- Cost
- Range
- Backup battery life

North Coast Medical Supply Catalog

www.BeAbleToDo.com

Search Terms
- Special utensils for eating
- Activities of daily living
- Hip problems
- Exercise and mobility
- EZ access

- Functional mobility
- Stability
- Personal care

Ohio State University Hearing Professionals

http://hearing.osu.edu/8590.cfm

Search Terms
- What is a hearing evaluation?
- Hearing aid care
- Payment for hearing aids

State Driving Laws

http://www.caring.com/calculators/state-driving-laws

Search Terms
- Specific rules for older drivers
- Vision test
- License renewal conditions

REFERENCES

American Ophthalmology Association (AOA). (2014). *Link for patients and the public—eye health at every age.* Retrieved April 26, 2014, from www.aoa.org

American Podiatric Medical Association (APMA). (2014). *Foot health.* Retrieved May 3, 2014, from http://www.apma.org/learn/FootHealthList.cfm?navItemNumber=498

Centers for Disease Control and Prevention (CDC). (2014). *Faststats: Inpatient surgery for the U.S.* Retrieved May 3, 2014, from http://www.cdc.gov/nchs/fastats/insurg.htm

Central Vermont Medical Center (CVMC). *Geriatric rehabilitation.* Retrieved May 3, 2014, from http://www.cvmc.org/hospital/departments-services/clinical-departments/rehabilitation-services/physical-therapy/geriatric-rehabilitation

Dewald, J. (2014). "Industrial Revolution." *Europe, 1450 to 1789: Encyclopedia of the early modern world. 2004. Encyclopedia.com*. Retrieved May 3, 2014, from http://www.encyclopedia.com/topic/Industrial_Revolution.aspx

Gheno, R., Cepparo, J., Rosca, C., & Cotton, A. (2012). Musculoskeletal disorders in the elderly. *Journal of Clinical Imaging Science, 2*, 39. Published online July 28, 2012. doi: 10.4103/2156–7514.99151. Retrieved May 1, 2014, from http://www.ncbi.nlm.nih.gov/pmc/articles/PMC3424705

Gross, M. (2010). Shoe wear recommendations for the older adult. *Clinical Geriatrics, 18*(5). Retrieved May 3, 2014, from http://www.clinicalgeriatrics.com/articles/Shoe-Wear-Recommendations-Older-Adult#sthash.DS5WyEPe.dpuf

LaBrasseour, N. (2014). *Slowing or reversing muscle loss. For medical professionals*. Mayo Clinic. Retrieved September 9, 2014, from HYPERLINK http://www.mayoclinic.org/medical-professionals/clinical-updates/physical-medicine-rehabilitatio (www.mayoclinic.org/medical-professionals/clinical-updates/physical-medicine-rehabilitation/slowing-or-reversing-muscle-loss)

Li-Korotky, H. -S. (2012). Age-related hearing loss: Quality of care for quality of life. *The Gerontologist, 52*(2), 265–271.

Mayo Clinic. (2014). *Muscle loss and aging: Mayo Clinic expert discusses strategies, therapies to restore muscle health*. Newswise. Retrieved May 1, 2014, from http://www.newswise.com/articles/muscle-loss-and-aging-mayo-clinic-expert-discusses-strategies-therapies-to-restore-muscle-health

McDaniel, K. (2012). Working and care-giving: The impact on caregiver stress, family-work conflict, and burnout *Journal of Life Care Planning, 10*(4), 21–32. Retrieved May 4, 2014, through Foley Center Library, CINAHL database, Gonzaga University from http://web.a.ebscohost.com.proxy.foley.gonzaga.edu/ehost/pdfviewer/pdfviewer?sid=2bf900b8–43e9–4757-8c5e-504a9760900a%40sessionmgr4003&vid=4&hid=4112

Menant, J., Perry, S., Steele, J., Menz, H., Munro, B., & Lord, S. (2008). Effects of shoe characteristics on dynamic stability when walking on even and uneven surfaces in young and older people. *Archives of Physical Medicine and Rehabilitation, 89*(10), 1970–1976.

National Institute on Aging/National Institutes of Health (NIA/NIH). (2014). *Health and aging—fatigue*. Retrieved May 3, 2014, from http://www.nia.nih.gov/health/topics/fatigue

Saczynski, J., & Rebok, G. (2004). Strategies for memory improvement in older adults. *Advanced Practice Nursing eJournal, 4*(1). Retrieved May 4, 2014, from http://www.medscape.com/viewarticle/465740

WebMD. (2012). *Aging well-healthy again—normal aging*. Retrieved April 24, 2014, from http://www.webmd.com/healthy-aging/tc/healthy-aging-normal-aging

WebMD. (2013). *Medications that can cause weakness or fatigue*. Retrieved May 3, 2014, from http://www.webmd.com/fibromyalgia/medications-that-can-cause-weakness-or-fatigue

Ziere, G., Dieleman, J. P., Hofman, A., Pols, H. A. P., van der Cammen, T. J. M., & Stricker, B. H. (2006). Polypharmacy and falls in the middle age and elderly population. *British Journal of Clinical Pharmacology, 61*(2), 218–223. Retrieved May 3, 2014, from http://www.ncbi.nlm.nih.gov/pmc/articles/PMC1885000

APPENDIX

Professional Foot Assessment

Client Name: _____ Date:_____

Diabetic: ___ YES ___NO

✓	Skin	Completed		Comments
	Lesions	LEFT	RIGHT	
	Fissures or open sores (circle)	LEFT	RIGHT	
	Corns or calluses	LEFT	RIGHT	
	Plantar wart	LEFT	RIGHT	
	Itching legs/feet	LEFT	RIGHT	
	Dry, flaky skin	LEFT	RIGHT	
	Rash	LEFT	RIGHT	
	Drainage	LEFT	RIGHT	
	Hair growth present	LEFT	RIGHT	
✓	**Toenails**	**Completed**		
	Ingrown or overgrown (circle)	LEFT	RIGHT	
	Thickened or broken (circle)	LEFT	RIGHT	
	Sides curling inward	LEFT	RIGHT	
	Discolored	LEFT	RIGHT	
	Missing (which?)	LEFT	RIGHT	
✓	**Appearance**	**Completed**		
	Bunion	LEFT	RIGHT	
	Hammer toe	LEFT	RIGHT	
	Swelling	LEFT	RIGHT	
✓	**Circulation**	**Completed**		
	Color_____ Temp_____	LEFT	RIGHT	
	Edema	LEFT	RIGHT	

Documentation Abbreviations

COLOR: PE (PALE): PK (PINK): R (RED): M (MOTTLED): D (DUSKY): B (BLACK)
TEMPERATURE: W (WARM); CL (COOL); CD (COLD)

6

Home-Style Adult Safety and Socialization Options

Brenda L. Bonham Howe

THE SIGNIFICANCE OF HOME-STYLE OPTIONS

When independence and safety are compromised, the next step is to consider how these needs may be met. This always means change at some level and it can be one of the most difficult transitions for an older person to face. Most older individuals want to remain in their own homes. The older population at this time were born between 1920 and 1945 with the baby boomers quickly approaching the geriatric age classification of 65 years and more (Administration on Aging [AOA], 2014). The generation born before 1945 is often referred to as the "radio babies" because their first experience with mass communication was by radio. Many of these people lived through the Great Depression and World War II. They learned to survive from a young age by carrying a part of the survival responsibility. Many grew up in rural areas where they awoke early to take care of farm chores. Going to school was often a luxury and many had to help harvest crops instead of attending school. This generation of individuals often presents a strong sense of independence and good old stubbornness. To take assistance from anyone may imply "taking handouts" or "taking charity," which goes against the values imbued during the depression years. In light of this, it is not too difficult to understand why many of these elderly individuals cling to their own home and memories (Rosenblatt, 2010). Another factor to consider when looking at housing and assistance options are the finances of the individual. Personal finances may be such that considering a move into some level of personal care facility is not possible without liquidating an existing estate.

If aging individuals are able to remain safely in their own homes, it is often best in many respects. They are usually more content and this helps to keep their psychological and emotional state at a healthier level with less inclination toward depression. Making a transition to another living arrangement can be very stressful and does magnify the sense of loss felt by the individual. Sometimes making the effort to try and support the person in his or her home environment is not successful. However, when adaptive measures prove to be not enough, it may help the individual to come to a point of acceptance that more help is needed for the sake of safety (National Academy on an Aging Society [NAAS], 2014).

HOME SAFETY INSPECTION

After evaluating the needs of the individual, possible solutions are considered. A safety assessment of the living environment is an important first step (Elder Care Team [ECT], 2012).

The assessment includes every area of the home from the entrances into and throughout the house. Many safety hazards may be reduced by removing small area rugs, clearing walking paths, installing hand rails where possible, including grab bars near the toilet and bathing area, improving the lighting, and decreasing the need to bend low or reach high by moving frequently used items into more convenient locations. Sometimes, ramps instead of steps can reduce fall risk and perhaps enable the person to be involved in church, senior centers, and other socialization venues. Decreased mobility contributes to being homebound and often lonely in addition to physical and mental decline.

Safety Inspectors

In some communities there may be individuals who provide home safety inspection as a public service. First, call the local fire department to see if they offer free safety inspections for seniors. Second, contact the local county health office and ask for the seniors and persons with disabilities department. They often keep brochures or business cards of people who provide services for others who are homebound or need other assistive support. Next, try the local senior center as they often maintain lists of contacts or even have volunteers who provide a variety of services for seniors. Finally, call the local home health agencies as they may also have a program where a therapist comes to the home and does a safety inspection as a public service. It is one way the therapist can also assess the person in the home and potentially educate the individual if some physical or occupational therapy may be of benefit. It is a marketing strategy for the agency when they provide the environmental safety assessment.

Remodel

The increasing need for aging Americans to remain in their homes has influenced new strategies for many architects and home builders. Many now advertise expertise in remodeling for the accessibility of individuals with limited mobility. The American Society of Interior Designers (ASID) has one design focus for active aging. Homes are built with the idea that the individuals will be able to remain in the home as they age, due to the universal function of the home design (ASID, 2012). The timing is right for the promotion of homes built with the ability to age in place as a sellable feature. Wide doors to accommodate wheelchairs are advantageous. Handicap accessible bathroom is a great feature and may serve the family or guests very well. Those are just a few of the changes that may enable an older person to remain in his or her own home longer.

IN-HOME CAREGIVER OPTIONS

When there is no available family member to step in and help a senior citizen in making decisions about additional care or support, there are several options to tap. Where to start depends on the current situation, that is, if the person is in the hospital or at home. Most hospitals have a utilization review process that begins from the time a person is admitted to the hospital. The utilization reviewer is a case manager who investigates the purpose of hospitalization and makes sure that the client receives the right care for the diagnosis (Stricker, 2010). A discharge planner is also assigned to follow the client and to work toward a smooth transition from the hospital back into the community. This is the point where the debility of the aging individual comes to light and concerns regarding safety must be addressed. The discharge planner will then collaborate with the physician and health care team to set up further evaluation and transition back into the community (Alper, O'Malley, & Greenwald, 2013).

If the individual is in his or her own home and demonstrates cognitive or physical decline, a primary care provider may order a home health evaluation, which is performed by a registered nurse (RN) or a physical therapist. This assessment can be the springboard to initiate additional in-home assistance or start the necessary process of transitioning to a safer environment. However, the length of time and amount of time that home health staff can spend in the home is limited (based on Medicare guidelines). Additional in-home help must come from other resources. Home health specifics are presented at length in Chapters 7 and 8.

Private Caregiver

Private-pay caregivers may be found through classified advertisements. Seniors and people with disabilities occasionally maintain a list of individuals who do private care. Private caregivers also may leave their business cards with home health agency patient care coordinators (Medicare-reimbursed agencies), because it may lead to work when the agency must discharge the client. When hiring a private caregiver, it is wise to check references and to inquire about their training and past experience. Check on liability concerns as well in the event the caregiver is injured in the home. Not all private caregivers carry their own liability insurance. Keep in mind that this is a high-turnover industry and hiring one individual may prove to not be a long-term solution.

Private Duty Home Care Agencies

Private duty or nonmedical home care agencies are one of the fastest growing options of health care in America (Tweed, 2010). These agencies are usually licensed, insured, and bonded, which relieves the homeowner of some liability issues. In addition, agencies maintain a number of employees (full time and part time) and can always arrange for a backup as needed. It is also one way to try out more than one caregiver in order to find a good personality fit between the client and the caregiver.

One advantage of the private duty agency over the medical home health agency is that the amount of time scheduled is solely up to the client and personal advocate. Some agencies do set a minimum limit of 4 hours, and others are a little more flexible. There is usually not a maximum number of hours, as the client is responsible for paying for the service contracted.

Private Duty Caregivers

Caregivers are trained in the basics of personal care. Some agencies may hire certified nursing assistants, individuals who have taken several weeks of standardized training and have passed a test given by the state board of nursing. These individuals are trained in taking vital signs, being alert to the nuances of potential skin breakdown, and recognition of changes that require immediate reporting to the agency nurse.

Home health aides (HHAs) often receive basic training through the agency. Duties revolve around activities of daily living (ADL); they assist with bathing, dressing, and combing hair, transferring to a wheelchair, or standing by when the client is walking.

Personal care assistants (PCAs) provide companionship and may provide light housekeeping duties such as laundry, ironing, meal preparation, and errands. In some agencies, the duties of a HHA and PCA overlap. It is important to clarify this with the agency. The level of experience provided by the agency will affect the hourly rate of the caregivers.

Licensed practical nurses (LPNs), licensed vocational nurses (LVNs), and RNs may also be on the private duty team. Hourly rates for nurses can run quite high (currently $50–$60 per hour). Services provided are usually limited to visitation and assessment, medication management, medication administration, coordination with the client's in-home care team (if applicable), communication with the primary care provider and pharmacy, and delegation of nursing tasks to the caregiver (American Nurses Association [ANA] & National Council of State Boards of Nursing [NCSBN], 2005; Trottier, 2014).

Changes in the client's health status may indicate a need for skilled medical care. The private duty nurse should contact the primary health care provider to request an order for a home health evaluation. It would be appropriate for the nurse to contact the client's family or medical power of attorney as well.

Licensing for Private Duty Home Care

Licensing for private duty home care businesses can vary from state to state. A website is provided at the end of this chapter, which connects with a 50-state survey of licensure requirements (Tweed, 2010).

DAY CARE

Thousands of adult day care facilities exist across the United States. The service is one that provides planned care supervision for less than 24 hours a day. These centers offer caregivers the ability to place their family members or clients in a safe, social environment when it is not safe to leave them at home without supervision. Short-term day care allows family caregivers time to shop, keep appointments, work away from home, and attend social functions.

Day services usually provide supervised and structured activities, meals, and personal care for functionally impaired adults. Some adult day services may offer individualized preventive, therapeutic, and restorative health-related services.

Staff and Training

The level of staff skill will vary according to the level of functional impairment accepted into the facility. Some adult day care limits clients to those who have the ability to do most of their ADL. On the other hand, facilities that accept clients with dementia or Alzheimer's are prepared to assist with toileting. Usually the staff requirements are not as stringent, unless they advertise as "day health" or "adult medical day care." When no health or medical services are advertised, facilities are not required to staff health care professionals. However, past work experience with the elderly would be an advantage. Memory care presents very unique challenges and specialized training is advisable. Some facilities utilize training videos that can be ordered through the Dementia Society of America and the Alzheimer's Society and other similar organizations. Many training videos are also available at the www.youtube.com website.

If the adult day care facility qualifies as a health care agency then their staff will include certified or licensed personnel and the agency will be able to bill insurance for covered services.

Licensure Requirements

Licensure expectations may vary from state to state, just as the definitions also vary. In some states, adult day care is identified as a community-based group program, nonresidential, and nonmedical, though attention to healthy living is expected. The key idea is that the clients are provided supportive care and supervision during their stay in the facility. Although some state guidelines specify the facilities are nonresidential, some exceptions are made in other states such that the same licensure will apply to an adult foster care home where the staff is willing to provide occasional respite day care.

A link is provided to a website where a state-by-state search may be done to review licensing guidelines.

GROUP HOMES

Group homes exist within many communities for the purpose of providing the elderly with assisted living benefits within a family-style setting. There are many variations in layout and design, because most are located in community neighborhoods populated by singles, couples, and families. The homes have been upgraded to meet state and county standards to ensure a safe environment for the residents. Some homes will have a visible name sign, but many simply blend with the neighborhood and just happen to have a wheelchair ramp instead of steps going up to the front door.

These group settings are known by several names and may also vary from state to state: residential care home, personal care home, adult foster care home, group home, guest home, room and board home, community-based alternatives (Medicaid), and assisted living home. Most of these homes are licensed to provide for one to six residents with a minimum of one caregiver present at all times.

Amenities

Each home is unique due to the variety of locations, structural style, interior layout, and decoration. Some homes have had modifications to the rooms and baths to incorporate safety features. Requirements for the homes may vary, too. Some homes are women only, men only, memory care, and some will require mobility without assistive devices. A small pet may be allowed by some, many will not allow smoking, and others may provide a safe outdoor garden for relaxation in fresh air. Some homes will allow family to bring in personal furnishings and decorations for the bedroom. Bathrooms may be en suite, though many group homes will provide one multiple use handicap accessible shower and commode.

The small venue of the group home enables the caregiver to encourage shared activities in the home-like setting. The living room is often the media room for television viewing or listening to music. The resident group is also small enough to be encouraged to engage in individual activities. Needlecraft work is common for those who still have the vision and finger dexterity. In some cases, the residents may still have the ability to help in the kitchen or do light-duty cleaning. This provides a sense of purpose for those who are able to take part in the everyday chores of home life (Assisted Living Center [ALC], 2014).

Licensure

Licensure is required in most states. Homes are licensed according to the level of care that the resident manager is qualified to provide.

The caregiver must possess the level of education and training to match the level of care.

Level 1, 2, or 3: Most states require this community-based type of care to follow strict guidelines for operation. All caregivers and home providers must have a certain level of training and experience in the care of seniors—the licensing level of the home dictates the level of experience required (Care Service Options [CSO], 2013).

Class I homes provide light care to people who need assistance with four or fewer ADL; residents must be in stable medical condition.

Class II homes provide moderate levels of care to people who need assistance in one or all of the six ADL.

Class III homes provide heavy levels of care to people who are dependent or who need a high level of assistance with four or more ADL. No more than one totally dependent person may be in the residence at one time (Multnomah County or Multco, 2014).

STAFF AND TRAINING

Most states require the caregivers to complete cardiopulmonary resuscitation (CPR) and first-aid classes. These may be completed at a community college, through a hospital education program, or at a chapter of the American Red Cross.

Provider training workshops are often initiated to ensure quality care or provide residential services in community settings, and are usually provided through the Department of Human Services, Seniors, and People with Disabilities in each state. Subjects covered include:

- Community residential services: the role of direct care staff
- The rights of individuals receiving mental health services
- Working with people: introduction to human needs, values, guiding principles, and effective teaching strategies
- Basic health and medication

- Nutrition and food services
- Environmental emergencies: preventing, preparing, and responding
- Working with people: positive techniques to address challenging behavior
- Advanced health and medication
- Responding to life-threatening situations: CPR and first-aid (Michigan Department of Community Health [MDCH], 2014)

Most states require annual continuing education for the caregivers in order to meet licensure renewal requirements. The number of education hours will vary by state (SCO, 2013).

SUMMARY

- Concern for safety is what often motivates research of optional living situations
- Most people want to remain in their home environment
- A home safety inspection is a good first step
- Remodeling the home with safety and access in mind may be beneficial
- In-home caregiver options may be considered: family member or private duty
- Licensure of private duty home care options
- Day care staff, education, and licensure
- Group home staff, education, and licensure

RESOURCES

Adult Day Care Organization

http://www.adultdaycare.org/directory

Search Terms
- Adult day care directory by state
- Are private day cares safe?

- How well trained are the staff?
- Parenting your parent
- You deserve time off

Alzheimer's

http://www.alz.org

Search Terms
- Alzheimer's and dementia
- In my area
- Education and resource center
- Life with ALZ

Collaborative Housing for 55+ H.E.A.R.T. Homes

http://www.elderhomeoptions.com

Search Terms
- Mission statement
- Services

Dementia

http://www.dementia.org

Search Terms
- Lewy body syndrome
- Early onset dementia
- Secondary dementia
- Dealing with violent behavior
- Treatment

Golden Girl Homes, Inc.

www.goldengirlhomes.us

Search Terms
- Available housing
- Did you know?

Guide to Home Care Licensure by State

http://www.privatedutytoday.com/guides/licensing/index.htm

Search Terms
- Caregiver quality assurance program
- Business start-up
- Policy and procedure manual

Respite Care

http://www.eldercare.gov/ELDERCARE.NET/Public/Resources/Factsheets/Respite_Care.aspx

Search Terms
- What is respite?
- How do you pay?
- How can I ensure quality care?

REFERENCES

Administration on Aging (AOA). (2014). *Aging statistics*. Department of Health and Human Services. Retrieved March 26, 2014, from http://www.aoa.gov/AoARoot/Aging_Statistics/index.aspx

Alper, E., O'Malley, T., & Greenwald, J. (2013). *Appropriateness for discharge*. UpToDate, Wolters—Kluwer. Retrieved March 29, 2014, from http://www.uptodate.com/contents/hospital-discharge?topicKey=PC%2F2790&elapsedTimeMs=5&view=print&displayedView=full

American Nurses Association (ANA) & National Council of State Boards of Nursing (NCSBN). (2005). *Joint statement on delegation*. Retrieved March 29 2014, from http://www.emergingrnleader.com/wp-content/uploads/2012/06/Delegation_joint_statement_NCSBN-ANA.pdf

American Society of Interior Designers (ASID). (2012). *Design for active aging*. Retrieved March 23, 2014, from http://www.asid.org/content/design-active-aging

Assisted Living Center (ALC). (2014). *Assisted living activities*. Retrieved April 5, 2014, from http://www.assistedlivingcenter.com/articles/assisted-living-activities

Care Service Options (CSO). (2013). *Adult foster care homes*. Retrieved April 5, 2014, from http://www.careserviceoptions.com/adult-foster-care-homes

Elder Care Team (ECT). (2012). *Senior home safety assessment*. Retrieved March 28, 2014, from http://www.eldercareteam.com/public/390.cfm

Michigan Department of Community Health (MDCH). (2014). *Training: Providing residential services in community settings training manual*. Retrieved April 6, 2014, from http://www.michigan.gov/mdch/0,1607,7-132-2941_4868_4899-174577--,00.html

Multnomah County or Multco. (2014). *Aging and disability services*. Retrieved April 6, 2014, from http://www.co.multnomah.or.us/ads/achp/publications/forms/class-ws.pdf

National Academy on an Aging Society (NAAS) (2014). *Links to selected online resources*. Retrieved March 29, 2014, from http://www.agingsociety.org/agingsociety/links/links_living.html

Rosenblatt, C. (2010). *Helping aging parents who don't want help*. Forbes. Retrieved March 29, 2014, from http://www.forbes.com/2010/09/15/helping-elderly-homecare-assisted-living-personal-finance-helping-aging-parents.html

Stricker, P. (2010). *The role of utilization management in case management*. Case Management Society of America (CMSA). Retrieved March 29, 2014, from http://www.cmsa.org/Individual/NewsEvents/HealthTechnologyArticles/tabid/649/Default.aspx

Trottier, L. (2014). *Your first hiring decision: Agency versus independent*. Caring.com. Retrieved March 29, 2014, from http://www.caring.com/articles/hiring-independently-or-via-agency

Tweed, S. (2010). *Guides to home care licensing in your state*. Private Duty Today: Tweed Jeffries Company. Retrieved March 29, 2014, from http://www.privatedutytoday.com/guides/licensing/index.htm

7

Home Health Services

Brenda L. Bonham Howe

HOME CARE IN THE UNITED STATES

Nursing care in the home environment can be documented from at least the 11th century (Marrelli, 1997). Medicare (federal) and Medicaid (state) were legislated in 1965 and have been powerful forces in the growth and structure of home care. In 1963, there were 1,100 home care programs. Due to the 1965 federally financed home health care program, Medicare became the basis for financial support and made health care services available to a segment of society previously not served (Marrelli, 1997).

Expansion of health services for the larger client base increased health care costs. In an effort to control the rising costs, systems of prospective payment were necessary. In the early 1980s, the Reagan administration initiated several changes to Social Security benefits. At that time, the Medicare outlays for hospital bills had increased more rapidly than payroll tax revenues. Federal Medicare expenditures had more than doubled between 1970 and 1980. Several factors were cited for this increase: an increase in the aging population, new diagnostic and treatment technologies, an excessive use of new technologies, and a concern that doctors and hospitals were enhancing revenue by ordering unnecessary tests and treatments (Jansson, 2001, pp. 293–299).

By 1985, hospital leaders looked toward many changes in policies and practice. Congress established standardized national levels of payment for 467 specific diagnoses also called diagnosis-related groups (DRGs). This meant that Medicare reimbursed hospitals by a predetermined fee for hospitalization, based on their diagnosis. It did not matter when the person was admitted or discharged. If the individual developed complications due to the treatment or surgery, the predetermined fee remained the same (Jansson, 2001). In a domino-like effect, hospitals added discharge planners or case managers to begin the client discharge plan on the day the individual was admitted to the hospital. Case managers tracked daily status to make sure clients were recovering and were discharged efficiently.

Individuality often becomes a hurdle on the road to standardization. The fact that not all people recuperate from illness or surgery at the same time means that not everyone is capable of returning to his or her usual environment as soon as the health care facility would prefer. The elderly or immune compromised are at risk of inadequate care in the transition from facility to facility or to their own home. This problem was recognized at the onset of the DRG changes that came about in 1986. Hospitals that did not have their own home health or hospice services considered adding the transitional services. Entrepreneurs saw this as an opportunity for establishing private or not-for-profit home care agencies.

Definition of Home Care Nursing Practice

Several professional groups have defined home care practice in an attempt to clarify standards that meet Medicare reimbursement guidelines:

- The American Medical Association (AMA) perceives all home care activities as those that are a logical extension of physician services.
- The American College of Physicians (ACP) defines home care as the provision of care in a patient's home rather than an institution or office.
- The American Hospital Association (AHA) lists particulars such as medical care and supervision, social work services, nursing and pharmaceutical services, as well as transportation and equipment.
- The American Nurses Association (ANA) defines the scope and distinguishing characteristics of home health care in its effort to define the practice. New scope and definitions were initiated in 2007 due to the onset of pandemic warnings and the prospects of natural and man-made disasters; the home and community are increasing in importance as the recommended point of care delivery. In the future, home health nurses may be called upon to coordinate and deliver care like never before.

Home health nursing practice focuses on providing quality health care for patients where a patient resides, whether a private home or an assisted living or personal care facility. The goal is to provide services and education to improve the client's function in order to live as independently as possible in a safe environment (Ellenbecker, Samia, Cushman, & Alster, 2008).

As a specialized area of community health nursing, this multidisciplinary specialty provides the full range of health care services for acute, chronic, or terminal illnesses to patients, their families, and other caregivers. Clients and caregivers are the foci of care. The goal is to initiate, manage, and evaluate resources necessary to promote an optimal level of well-being.

The National Association of Home Care (NAHC) definition includes services to people who are recovering, disabled, chronically ill, or who may be in danger of abuse or neglect. Generally, it defines care that cannot be easily or effectively provided by informal caregivers for any length of time (NAHC, 2013).

The Centers for Disease Control and Prevention (CDC, 2012) definition is the most comprehensive and states that home health care "is provided to individuals and families in their places of residence for the purpose of promoting, maintaining, or restoring health or for maximizing the level of independence while minimizing the effects of disability and illness, including terminal illness." Services are based on admission assessment and are individualized to the needs of the individual patient and his or her family. An agency that is certified to provide medically skilled services coordinates scheduled visits by the appropriate health care professionals.

CURRENT HOME CARE ORGANIZATIONS

There are five categories of home care agencies based on their mission, vision, and administrative and organizational framework. The managed care environment has also impelled some agencies to merge or form coalitions. For instance, a hospital may merge with a nonprofit home health and hospice agency in order to provide care across a defined geographic area.

Official Home Care Agencies

Official home care agencies are nonprofit entities that have the support of public funding and qualify for Medicare and Medicaid reimbursement as well as from private payers (Centers for Medicare and Medicaid Services [CMS], 2012). A county or other municipal health department is an example of an official home care agency (DCHS, 2014). Many municipal health departments function as a resource for information about networking with other agencies. Some of the community services offered may include licensing for child care and adult foster care, reproductive health clinics, tuberculosis testing and follow-up, and aging and disability services.

Some agencies have funding for nurse case managers, but their role is more of coordinating necessary services by communication with the health care provider and other agencies.

Voluntary and Private Nonprofit Agencies

These agencies are supported by community-based charities, private donations, and by reinvesting the earnings and reserves of the business. They may also be approved for billing Medicare, Medicaid, and private insurances. The governing bodies often serve on a board of members from the community who volunteer leadership and expertise. The organizations are accountable to the communities and populations they serve. A private nonprofit agency must apply to the Internal Revenue Service (IRS) for tax-exempt status. To qualify, applicants must complete and submit the IRS Form 1023.

Combination

Agencies can be a combination of the official and the voluntary. For example, an official home health agency may form a business with a nonprofit hospice service.

Hospital-Based Home Health Agencies

A hospital-based home health agency shares the hospital's established board of directors. The transfer of inpatients to the hospital home-based service may provide a level of continuity of care that would not be experienced by the transfer to another agency. The additional service of home health care generates additional revenue for the hospital.

Proprietary Agencies

Proprietary agencies are privately owned and are not eligible for tax exemption. These agencies are run for the profit of the owners and the owners are responsible for all aspects of administration (Merriam-Webster Online, 2013).

WHAT DOES MEDICARE-APPROVED HOME HEALTH PROVIDE?

Home health care provides medical treatment for an illness or injury, with the goal of helping the client recover, regain independence, and become as self-sufficient as possible. More than just providing excellent care in the home, home health care also saves billions of dollars each year. These are the most cost-effective providers of health care in our country (Esposito, 2009; Wieberg, 2011).

REGULATORY AGENCIES

In 1965, Medicare was authorized under Title XVIII of the Social Security Act as a two-part (A and B) federal program for people who are 65 years and older, or disabled, or have end-stage renal disease (ESRD; Tables 7.1 and 7.2). As the world's largest health insurance program there are coverage rules and exclusions to coverage and eligibility (Social Security Administration [SSA], 2013). Medicare has developed many of the standards related to home care. Because Medicare is a health insurance program, the first requirement for home health service is that the client must have a medical problem. Agencies that qualify for Medicare reimbursement for services given must adhere consistently to the regulations set by the CMS (CMS, 2014). Regulatory agency inspectors who review policy and procedure manuals in addition to client records make periodic unannounced visits. The inspector may ride along with various staff members as they make home client visits.

The CMS is a federal agency within the U.S. Department of Health and Human Services (USDHHS) that manages the Medicare program and works in tandem with state government agencies to administer Medicaid, the State Children's Health Insurance

TABLE 7.1
Medicare Coverage Is Based on Three Primary Factors

- Federal and state laws
- National coverage decisions made by Medicare about whether something is covered
- Local coverage decisions made by companies in each state that process claims for Medicare. These companies decide whether something is medically necessary and should be covered in their area.

Source: CMS (2014).

Program (SCHIP), and health insurance portability standards. In addition to these programs, the CMS has other responsibilities, including the administrative simplification standards from the Health Insurance Portability and Accountability Act of 1996 (HIPAA; Marrelli, 1997).

Medicare Conditions of Participation

The CMS develops, reviews, and updates conditions of participation (CoPs) and conditions for coverage (CfCs; Table 7.3). Health care organizations must meet the CMS standards in order to begin and continue participating in the Medicare and Medicaid programs. The purpose of these health and safety standards is improvement of quality and protection of the health and safety of beneficiaries. The CMS also ensures that the standards of accrediting organizations recognized by the CMS (through a process called "deeming") meet or exceed the Medicare standards set forth in the CoPs/CfCs.

To further clarify, for a health care organization to participate in and receive payment from Medicare or Medicaid, it must meet the eligibility requirements for participation, which include a certificate of compliance with the CoPs or CfCs (CfCs for health care suppliers) as defined by federal regulations. The certification is awarded following a survey conducted by a state agency on behalf of the CMS. The Joint Commission (TJC) regulations state, "[h]owever, if

TABLE 7.2
Medicare Part A and B Coverage

Medicare A provides funding for covered inpatient hospitalization and skilled nursing facility (SNF) stays, with the patient having some financial responsibility in the form of deductibles.
(*Medicare and You Handbook*) www.medicare.gov/Pubs/pdf/10050.pdf

What does Medicare Part A cover?
- Inpatient care in hospitals
- Inpatient care in skilled nursing facilities (not custodial or long-term care)
- Hospice care services
- Home health care services
- Inpatient care in a religious nonmedical health care institution

www.medicare.gov/Pubs/pdf/10050.pdf

What does Medicare Part B cover?
Medicare Part B covers two types of services
- Preventive services; health care to prevent illness (such as flu or pneumonia vaccine)
- Medically necessary services
  - Services or supplies that are needed to diagnose or treat a person's medical condition and that meet accepted standards of medical practice (ostomy supplies, durable medical equipment, etc.). If these supplies are obtained through a health care provider who accepts "assignment," then the person qualified for Medicare Part B does not owe any money out-of-pocket. Assignment refers to an agreement made by a doctor, other health care provider, or a supplier that they will be paid directly by Medicare and will accept the payment amount set by Medicare. In turn, the provider will not bill the client for more than the Medicare deductible and coinsurance.
- Part B will cover:
  - Ambulance services
  - Clinical research
  - Durable medical equipment (DME)
  - Getting a second opinion before surgery
  - Inpatient services
  - Limited outpatient prescriptions
  - Mental health
  - Outpatient services

There are services that Medicare does not cover. It is important for individuals to review what Medicare coverage is best for them and to consider a complementary supplemental insurance.

Some of the items and services that Medicare does not cover include:
- Acupuncture
- Cosmetic surgery
- Dentures
- Hearing aids and fitting examinations
- Long-term care (custodial care)
- Routine dental or eye care

Source: CMS (2014).

TABLE 7.3
CoPs and CfCs Apply to the Following Health Care Organizations

Ambulatory surgical centers (ASCs)
Comprehensive outpatient rehabilitation facilities (CORFs)
Critical access hospitals (CAHs)
End-stage renal disease facilities
Federally qualified health centers
Home health agencies
Hospices
Hospitals
Hospital swing beds
Intermediate care facilities for individuals with intellectual disabilities (ICF/IID)
Organ procurement organizations (OPOs)
Portable x-ray suppliers
Programs for all-inclusive care for the elderly organizations (PACE)
Clinics, rehabilitation agencies, and public health agencies as providers of outpatient physical therapy and speech–language pathology services
Psychiatric hospitals
Religious nonmedical health care institutions
Rural health clinics
Long-term care facilities
Transplant centers

CfCs, conditions for coverage; CoPs, conditions of participation.
Source: CMS (2014).

a national accrediting organization, such as The Joint Commission, has and enforces standards that meet or exceed Medicare's CoPs (or CfCs), CMS may grant the accrediting organization 'deeming' authority" (TJC, 2012a).

The Joint Commission

TJC is an independent, not-for-profit organization that grew out of a grassroots movement in 1910 when Ernest Codman, MD, proposed an "end result system of hospital standardization." Under this system, Dr. Codman proposed that hospitals track patients long enough to determine if the treatment had been effective. If symptoms had not resolved, then staff physicians would attempt to identify further treatment. By performing these standards, they hoped to improve treatment outcomes in the future. The system proved so effective over the years that TJC was founded in 1951 and now accredits and certifies more than 20,000 health care organizations and programs in the United States. Accreditation and certification by TJC are recognized nationwide as a symbol of excellence that reflects an organization's commitment to meet high performance standards (TJC, 2013b).

QUALIFICATIONS FOR HOME HEALTH SERVICE

Skilled Medical Care

Medicare covers "medically necessary" part-time or intermittent skilled nursing care and/or physical therapy, and possibly assistance from other members of the home health team. A doctor, or a health care provider who works with a doctor, must see the potential home health client face to face so that he or she can certify the need for home health service. In most states, a doctor must order the home health care and a Medicare-certified home health agency must provide it. Medicare also requires a homebound status for the client. Some clients would decline home health service because they do not wish to comply with the homebound guidelines. From the Medicare perspective, if a person is able to drive or commute without considerable or taxing effort, then it is possible for the individual to obtain outpatient services (Murtaugh, 2013).

Homebound

Another condition to which some potential clients object is that the individual is to be "homebound." The term itself may alarm potential clients. However, what is meant is that the health status currently interferes with the individual's normal ability to leave the house. Trips away from home require considerable and taxing effort from the client. Furthermore, trips away from home are brief and infrequent. Otherwise, the individual would be capable of medical outpatient visits, which would not require the level of reimbursement necessary for home health service.

Typical reasons why leaving home would be a painstaking effort include the use of mobility equipment, diminished function in an upper or lower extremity, restricted mobility due to pain or weakness, and symptoms of severe cardiovascular disease. There are certain situations when outings are considered permissible and they are at the discretion of the client and caregiver: religious services, family reunions, funerals, graduations, and medical appointments. Potential clients who feel that they cannot limit their outings may prefer to forego home health service. When that situation occurs, the home health representative who made the initial visit will have to notify the referring health care provider so that outpatient visits can be arranged.

SERVICES PROVIDED BY HOME HEALTH TEAM MEMBERS

Shared Responsibilities

All home health team members must be attentive to multilevel communication that is necessary to ensure continuity and quality of care. Effective communication is vital among the home health team member, the client, and key family or friends. Coordination with the physician is imperative for client updates and to acquire new orders or discontinue old orders. The home health team members must communicate with each other to update on any client status changes or changes made to the plan of care. To complete the circle of communication, the information is relayed back to the client and personal caregivers. Without a complete circle of communication, something will fall through the cracks and that cannot only be dangerous, but can also impact the reputation of the organization.

Each team member plays the role of an educator at some point in his or her home health work. The primary information revolves around the client's treatment regimen. Clients and caregivers are included in the creation of the plan of care. It is important for them to "buy into" the plan or the goals that were set may never be reached.

All home health team members are aware of the Fall Intervention Program for clients (Williams, 2007). It is every team member's role to teach and reinforce safe practices at home to avoid injury. A concern for fall risk increases with older clients. Falls contribute to injuries, hospitalization, loss of independence, and sometimes death. Medicare has published guidelines for a fall risk program, which is utilized by all federally supported agencies. Home health agencies strive to improve the client's health and to avoid cause for rehospitalization. Medicare tracks episodes of rehospitalizations and readmission to home health services in order to study potential means for improved outcomes. Medicare's Bundling Pilot: Including Post-Acute Care Services is in effect as of 2013 (Dummit, 2011).

Home health team members also attend and contribute to weekly or bimonthly case conferences and other meetings as required by the organization policy to ensure coordinated and comprehensive plans of care for the patients of the organization. Discussion also includes a review of patient and family/caregiver needs for other home health disciplines and referrals as appropriate.

Last, but not least, all team members are responsible for completing, submitting, and synchronizing all client documentation and clinical notes including Medicare's Outcome and Assessment Information Set (OASIS) within 24 hours of discharge (Partners in Care Home Health & Hospice [PIC], 2013).

OUTCOME AND ASSESSMENT INFORMATION SET

Patients are dependent on accurate assessment and documentation of their health care needs. If documentation does not support the services being given, then Medicare or Medicaid may deny coverage of all or part of the home care support (see the Appendix to this chapter).

JOB DESCRIPTIONS

Registered Nurse

Job Description

The registered nurse plans, coordinates, implements, and evaluates home health and hospice services, and is experienced in nursing, with an emphasis on community health education. The professional nurse builds from the resources of the organization and community to provide services to meet the needs of individuals and families within their homes. The registered nurse is responsible for cost-efficient and effective patient care with quality outcomes. Registered nurses may work under several different job titles in a home health setting. These various roles and competency requirements are discussed in Chapter 8: "Skilled Nurse Competency Requirements for Home Health Services."

Home Health Aide

Job Description

The home health aide (HHA) is a paraprofessional member of the interdisciplinary team who works under the supervision of a registered nurse or therapist. The aide practices within the scope of practice defined by the State Board of Nursing and adheres to the plan of care. The aide is responsible for observing the patient and documenting and reporting to the care manager the patient's status.

Essential Job Functions

The responsibilities of the HHA include, but are not limited to, the following.

- Provides personal care as outlined in the plan of care, maintaining patient privacy
- Provides extension of therapy services by assistance in ambulation or exercise as delegated by the therapist and outlined in the plan of care
- Takes vital signs and communicates changes/concerns as outlined on the plan of care to the care manager
- Assesses pain using the organization's pain scale and reports to the care manager per the plan of care
- Observes patient's skin and provides appropriate care to prevent breakdown of tissue
- Reports any changes in a patient's condition to the care manager
- Assists with other tasks and duties as outlined in the plan of care and scope of practice and as delegated or assigned by the registered nurse or therapist

Effective August 14, 1990, an HHA must have successfully completed a state-established or other training program that meets the requirements of S 484.36(a) and a competency evaluation program, or state licensure program that meets the requirements of S 484.36(b), or a competency evaluation program or state licensure program that meets the requirements of S 484.36(b).

The home health/hospice aide may perform certain functions when delegated by the registered nurse as outlined by the State Board of Nursing delegation rules (PIC, 2013).

Physical Therapist

Job Description

The physical therapist plans, coordinates, implements, and evaluates home health and hospice therapy services. The physical therapist is knowledgeable in providing therapy in the home setting. The therapist builds from the resources of the organization and community to provide services to meet the needs of individuals and families within their homes. The physical therapist is responsible for cost-effective and effective patient care with quality outcomes.

Essential Job Functions

- Completes an initial comprehensive (if home health includes OASIS) and accurate assessment of client and family to determine home health needs
- Develops an individualized care plan, which establishes measurable goals based on the therapy assessment including the patient's functional abilities and limitations, rehabilitation potential, and diagnosis
- Initiates appropriate preventive and rehabilitation treatment and procedures
- Provides physical therapy instructions and health education protocol instructions to patient, family, and caregivers as appropriate
- Adapts teaching styles to meet patient and family needs
- Ensures that arrangements for equipment and other necessary items and services are available and provided
- Identifies discharge planning needs as part of the care plan development and implements these prior to discharge of the patient (PIC, 2013)

Occupational Therapist

Job Description

The occupational therapist, contracted or employed through the organization, is responsible for providing occupational therapy services and for adhering to all state, federal, and compliance regulations.

Essential Job Functions

- Evaluates patient's functional status (muscle function, endurance, visual coordination, written and verbal communication skills, self-care ability, work capacity, etc.); evaluates the home environment for hazards or barriers to more independent living. Identifies equipment needs; participates in the development of the plan of care
- Develops the treatment program and establishes goals for improved function; communicates the plan of care to the referring physician and other clinicians involved in the patient's care
- Teaches new skills or retrains the patient in once-familiar daily activities that have been lost due to illness or injury
- Fabricates splints and instructs patients regarding the use of various types of adaptive equipment to improve function
- Trains the patient in the use of prosthetic and/or orthotic devices

Speech Therapist

Job Description

The speech–language pathologist is responsible for implementation of standards of care for speech–language pathology services and for adherence to all conditions in the service agreement.

Essential Job Functions

- Conducts appropriate evaluations, assesses home environment (as appropriate), and identifies equipment needs relative to speech/language function
- Identifies functional speech and swallow defects and establishes a plan of care to improve the patient's function
- Administers a speech therapy program using specialized therapeutic technique and/or equipment
- Recommends communication devices/aids as indicated
- Performs other duties as required to facilitate the delivery of speech–language pathology services (PIC, 2013)

Medical Social Worker

Job Description

The medical social worker provides counseling and related support services to assist in meeting the identified psychosocial needs of patients and families enrolled in home health or hospice services.

Essential Job Functions

- Completes comprehensive psychosocial assessments on patients/families referred for home services
- Contributes to the interdisciplinary plan of care by establishing goals and intervention based on patient/family psychosocial issues and needs identified in the assessment process
- Provides a range of professional social work services to refer appropriate patients/families to address identified needs including, but not limited to, ongoing assessment services, counseling, emotional support, home care planning, patient/

family education, resource identification, information and referral, advocacy, and other supportive services
- Collaborates with other departments such as transitions and volunteer services to assist in meeting identified needs of patients/families
- Assists in providing information, referral, and support services to community members seeking assistance
- Establishes and maintains collaborative relationships with related community agencies/resources to support patient/family care and identified psychosocial needs; promotes and assists with education and support activities to related community agencies/resources (PIC, 2013)

Registered Dietician

Job Description

Responsible for the assessment, intervention, and teaching of patients' complex nutritional needs relative to medical diagnosis.

Essential Job Functions

- Assesses patients' complex nutritional needs based on history, current diagnoses, and symptoms
- Develops an appropriate plan of care with the patient to meet nutritional goals; adapts the plan to suit the patient's ability, economic status, and lifestyle
- Provides appropriate counseling and education to the patient and family/caregiver regarding medical nutritional therapy including nutritional principles, dietary plans, food selection, and economics
- Evaluates the patient's progress toward nutritional goals and readjusts the plan of care as needed (PIC, 2013)

SUMMARY

- Home health service brings medical professional care to the individual, which helps reduce health care costs associated with hospital and skilled care facilities.
- Medicare reimburses eligible clients. However, not all home health agencies are eligible for Medicare reimbursement.
- Home health care is defined and standardized by several professional medical organizations to clarify Medicare reimbursement guidelines.
- Home care organizations include official home care, voluntary and private nonprofit, hospital based, and proprietary.
- Medicare follows specific guidelines as to what home care services and supplies are reimbursed to official home care agencies.
- Regulatory agencies oversee compliance standards of client care wherever Medicare reimbursement is provided.
- Health care agencies must meet Medicare CoPs to maintain licensure.
- Clients must meet specific qualifications for official home health service. This is determined with the use of an assessment guide developed by the CMS. The assessment is called OASIS.
- Home health professionals who provide in-home care include the registered nurse, HHA, physical therapist, occupational therapist, speech therapist, medical social worker, and registered dietician.

RESOURCE

National Association of Home Care & Hospice

www.nahc.org

Search Terms
- Mission
- Membership
- Education

REFERENCES

Centers for Disease Control and Prevention (CDC). (2012). *Home health definitions of terms.* Retrieved October 2013, from http://www.cdc.gov/nchs/nhhcs/nhhcs_home_highlights.htm

Centers for Medicare and Medicaid Services (CMS). (2014). *Conditions for coverage (CfCs) & conditions of participations (CoPs).* Retrieved from http://www.cms.gov/Regulations-and-Guidance/Legislation/CFCsAndCoPs/index.html

Deschutes County Health Department (DCHS). (2013). *Health services.* Retrieved from http://www.deschutes.org/Health-Services.aspx#

Dummit, L. (2011). *Medicare's bundling pilot-including post acute care services.* National Health Policy Forum. Issue brief #841. Retrieved October 20, 2013, from http://www.nhpf.org/library/issue-briefs/IB841_BundlingPostAcuteCare_03-28-11.pdf

Ellenbecker, C. H., Samia, L., Cushman, M. J., & Alster, K. (2008). *Patient safety and quality: An evidence-based handbook for nurses.* Rockville, MD: Agency for Healthcare Research and Quality (Chapter 13). Retrieved October 15, 2013, from http://www.ncbi.nlm.nih.gov/books/NBK2631

Esposito, L. (2009). *New report: Home health care saves billions for Medicare.* Retrieved October 2013 from http://www.congressweb.com/nahc/docfiles/march_on_wash_09/Avalere%20Study.pdf

Jansson, B. (2001). *The reluctant welfare state: American social welfare policies—past, present, and future.* Belmont, CA: Wadsworth/Thomson Learning.

Marrelli, T. M. (1997). *Handbook of home health orientation.* St. Louis, MO: Mosby Year Book, Inc.

Merriam-Webster Online. (2013). *Proprietary.* Retrieved October 20, 2013, from http://www.merriam-webster.com/dictionary/proprietary

Murtaugh, C. (2013). *Clarifying the definition of homebound and medical necessity using OASIS data: Final report.* U.S. Department of Health and Human Services Center for Home Care Policy and Research. Retrieved October 25, 2013, from http://aspe.hhs.gov/daltcp/reports/OASISfr.pdf

National Association of Home Care & Hospice. (2013). Hospice facts and statistics. Retrieved July 4, 2014 from www.nahc.org

Partners in Care Home Health & Hospice (PIC). (2013). *Health professionals job descriptions*. Used by permission of Kenneth Koenig, Human Resources Director. Bend, Oregon.

Social Security Administration (SSA). (2013). *History of SSA during the Johnson administration 1963–1968*. Retrieved October 31, 2013, from www.ssa.gov/history/ssa/lbjmedicare1.html

The Joint Commission (TJC). (2012). *Facts about federal deemed status and state recognition*. Retrieved October 26, 2013, from http://www.jointcommission. org/assets/1/18/Facts_about_Federal_Deemed_Status1.PDF

The Joint Commission (TJC). (2013a). *Joint commission history*. Retrieved October 20, 2013, from http://www.jointcommission.org/assets/1/6/Joint_Commission_History.pdf

The Joint Commission (TJC). (2013b). *About the Joint Commission*. Retrieved October 20, 2013, from http://www.jointcommission.org/about_us/about_the_joint_commission_main.aspx

Wieberg, D. (2011). *New study sees growing home health care as key to saving U.S. billions in hospital costs*. PRNewswire. Retrieved October 15, 2013, from http://www.prnewswire.com/news-releases/new-study-sees-growing-home-health-care-as-key-to-saving-us-billions-in-hospital-costs-114144914.html

Williams, L. (2007). Liability landscape: Are your fall interventions enough? *Nursing Home Magazine*, October 1, 2007. Retrieved October 31, 2013, from http://www.thefreelibrary.com/Are+your+fall+interventions+enough%3F-a0171889735

APPENDIX

According to the Paperwork Reduction Act of 1995, no persons are required to respond to a collection of information unless it displays a valid Office of Management and Budget (OMB) control number. The valid OMB control number for this information collection instrument is 0938-0760. The time required to complete this information collection is estimated to average 0.7 minutes per response, including the time to review instructions, search existing data resources, gather the data needed, and complete and review the information collection. If you have comments concerning this form, please write to: CMS, 7500 Security Boulevard, Attn: PRA Reports Clearance Officer, Baltimore, Maryland 21244-1850.

HOME HEALTH PATIENT TRACKING SHEET

(M0010) CMS Certification Number: __ __ __ __
(M0014) Branch State: __ __
(M0016) Branch ID Number: __ __ __ __ __ __ __ __
(M0018) National Provider Identifier (NPI) for the attending physician who has signed the plan of care: __ __ __ __ __ __ __ __ __ __ ☐ UK – Unknown or Not Available
(M0020) Patient ID Number: __ __ __ __ __ __ __ __ __ __ __ __
(M0030) Start of Care [SOC] Date: __ __ / __ __ / __ __
            month / day / year
(M0032) Resumption of Care [ROC] Date: __ __ / __ __ / __ __ __ __
☐ NA – Not Applicable   month / day / year
(M0040) Patient Name: _____
        (First)   (MI)   (Last)   (Suffix)
(M0050) Patient State of Residence: ____
(M0060) Patient Zip Code: _____

(M0063)   Medicare Number: __ __ __ __ __ __ __ __ __ __ __ __
          ☐ NA – No Medicare   (including suffix)
(M0064)   Social Security Number:__ __ __ - __ __ - __ __ __ __
          ☐ UK – Unknown or Not Available
(M0065)   Medicaid Number: __ __ __ __ __ __ __ __ __ __ __ __
          ☐ NA – No Medicaid
(M0066)   Birth Date: __ __ / __ __ / __ __
                      month/day/year
(M0069)   Gender:
          ☐ 1 - Male
          ☐ 2 - Female

(M0140)   Race/Ethnicity: (Mark all that apply.)
          ☐ 1 - American Indian or Alaska Native
          ☐ 2 - Asian
          ☐ 3 - Black or African American
          ☐ 4 - Hispanic or Latino
          ☐ 5 - Native Hawaiian or Pacific Islander
          ☐ 6 - White

(M0150)   Current Payment Sources for Home Care: (Mark all that apply.)
          ☐ 0 - None; no charge for current services
          ☐ 1 - Medicare (traditional fee-for-service)
          ☐ 2 - Medicare (HMO/managed care/advantage plan)
          ☐ 3 - Medicaid (traditional fee-for-service)
          ☐ 4 - Medicaid (HMO/managed care)
          ☐ 5 - Workers' compensation
          ☐ 6 - Title programs (e.g., Title III, V, or XX)
          ☐ 7 - Other government (e.g., TriCare, VA, etc.)
          ☐ 8 - Private insurance
          ☐ 9 - Private HMO/managed care
          ☐ 10 - Self-pay
          ☐ 11 - Other (specify) _____
          ☐ UK - Unknown

OUTCOME AND ASSESSMENT INFORMATION SET

Items to be Used at Specific Time Points

Start of Care Start of care—further visits planned	M0010-M0030, M0040-M0150, M1000-M1036, M1100-M1242, M1300-M1302, M1306, M1308-M1324, M1330-M1350, M1400, M1410, M1600-M1730, M1740-M1910, M2000, M2002, M2010, M2020-M2250
Resumption of Care Resumption of care (after inpatient stay)	M0032, M0080-M0110, M1000-M1036, M1100-M1242, M1300-M1302, M1306, M1308-M1324, M1330-M1350, M1400, M1410, M1600-M1730, M1740-M1910, M2000, M2002, M2010, M2020-M2250
Follow-Up Recertification (follow-up) assessment Other follow-up assessment	M0080-M0100, M0110, M1020-M1030, M1200, M1242, M1306, M1308, M1322-M1324, M1330-M1350, M1400, M1610, M1620, M1630, M1810-M1840, M1850, M1860, M2030, M2200
Transfer to an Inpatient Facility Transferred to an inpatient facility—patient not discharged from an agency Transferred to an inpatient facility—patient discharged from agency	M0080-M0100, M1040-M1055, M1500, M1510, M2004, M2015, M2300-M2410, M2430-M2440, M0903, M0906
Discharge From Agency— Not to an Inpatient Facility	
Death at Home	M0080-M0100, M0903, M0906

Discharge From Agency	M0080-M0100, M1040-M1055, M1230, M1242, M1306-M1350, M1400-M1620, M1700-M1720, M1740, M1745, M1800-M1890, M2004, M2015-M2030, M2100-M2110, M2300-M2420, M0903, M0906

CLINICAL RECORD ITEMS

(M0080) Discipline of Person Completing Assessment:
☐ 1-RN ☐ 2-PT ☐ 3-SLP/ST ☐ 4-OT

(M0090) Date Assessment Completed: __ __ / __ __ / __ __
                                                        month / day / year

(M0100) This Assessment Is Currently Being Completed for the Following Reasons

Start/Resumption of Care
☐ 1 – Start of care—further visits planned
☐ 3 – Resumption of care (after inpatient stay)
Follow-Up
☐ 4 – Recertification (follow-up) reassessment [*Go to M0110*]
☐ 5 – Other follow-up [*Go to M0110*]
Transfer to an Inpatient Facility
☐ 6 – Transferred to an inpatient facility—patient not discharged from agency [*Go to M1040*]
☐ 7 – Transferred to an inpatient facility—patient discharged from agency [*Go to M1040*]
Discharge From Agency—Not to an Inpatient Facility
☐ 8 – Death at home [*Go to M0903*]
☐ 9 – Discharge from agency [*Go to M1040*]

(M0102) **Date of Physician-Ordered SOC (ROC):** If the physician indicated a specific start of care (resumption of care) date when the patient was referred for home health services, record the date specified.

__ __ / __ __ / __ __ [*Go to M0110, if date entered*]
month / day / year

☐ NA – No specific SOC date ordered by physician

(M0104) **Date of Referral:** Indicate the date that the written or verbal referral for initiation or resumption of care was received by the HHA.

__ __ / __ __ / __ __
month / day / year

(M0110) **Episode Timing:** Is the Medicare home health payment episode for which this assessment will define a case mix group an "early" episode or a "later" episode in the patient's current sequence of adjacent Medicare home health payment episodes?

☐ 1 - Early
☐ 2 - Later
☐ UK - Unknown
☐ NA - Not Applicable: No Medicare case mix group to be defined by this assessment

PATIENT HISTORY AND DIAGNOSES

(M1000) From which of the following **Inpatient Facilities** was the patient discharged *during the past 14 days*? **(Mark all that apply.)**

☐ 1 - Long-term nursing facility (NF)
☐ 2 - Skilled nursing facility (SNF/TCU)
☐ 3 - Short-stay acute hospital (IPPS)
☐ 4 - Long-term care hospital (LTCH)

☐ 5 - Inpatient rehabilitation hospital or unit (IRF)
☐ 6 - Psychiatric hospital or unit
☐ 7 - Other (specify)
☐ NA - Patient was not discharged from an inpatient facility [*Go to M1016*]

(M1005) **Inpatient Discharge Date** (most recent):
__ __ / __ __ / __ __
month / day / year
☐ UK - Unknown

(M1010) List each **Inpatient Diagnosis** and ICD-10-CM code at the level of highest specificity for only those conditions treated during an inpatient stay within the past 14 days (no E-codes or V-codes):

Inpatient Facility Diagnosis	ICD-10-CM Code
a.	
b.	
c.	
d.	
e.	
f.	

(M1012) List each **Inpatient Procedure** and the associated ICD-10-CM procedure code relevant to the plan of care.

Inpatient Procedure	Procedure Code
a.	
b.	
c.	
d.	

☐ NA - Not applicable
☐ UK - Unknown

(M1016) **Diagnoses Requiring Medical or Treatment Regimen Change Within Past 14 Days:** List the patient's **Medical Diagnoses** and ICD-10-CM codes at the level of highest specificity for those conditions requiring changed medical or treatment regimen within the past 14 days (no surgical, E-codes, or V-codes):

Changed Medical Regimen Diagnosis	ICD-10-CM Code
a. _____	___ ___ ___ . ___ ___ ___
b. _____	___ ___ ___ . ___ ___ ___
c. _____	___ ___ ___ . ___ ___ ___
d. _____	___ ___ ___ . ___ ___ ___
e. _____	___ ___ ___ . ___ ___ ___
f. _____	___ ___ ___ . ___ ___ ___

☐ NA - Not applicable (no medical or treatment regimen changes within the past 14 days)

(M1018) **Conditions Prior to Medical or Treatment Regimen Change or Inpatient Stay Within Past 14 Days**: If this patient experienced an inpatient facility discharge or change in medical or treatment regimen within the past 14 days, indicate any conditions which existed *prior to* the inpatient stay or change in medical or treatment regimen. **(Mark all that apply.)**

☐ 1 - Urinary incontinence
☐ 2 - Indwelling/suprapubic catheter
☐ 3 - Intractable pain
☐ 4 - Impaired decision making
☐ 5 - Disruptive or socially inappropriate behavior
☐ 6 - Memory loss to the extent that supervision required
☐ 7 - None of the above

☐ NA - No inpatient facility discharge *and* no change in medical or treatment regimen in past 14 days
☐ UK - Unknown

(M1020/ 1022/ 1024) **Diagnoses, Symptom Control, and Payment Diagnoses:** List each diagnosis for which the patient is receiving home care (Column 1) and enter its ICD-10-CM code at the level of highest specificity (no surgical/procedure codes) (Column 2). Diagnoses are listed in the order that best reflects the seriousness of each condition and supports the disciplines and services provided. Rate the degree of symptom control for each condition (Column 2). Choose one value that represents the degree of symptom control appropriate for each diagnosis: V-codes (for M1020 or M1022) or E-codes (for M1022 only) may be used. ICD-10-CM sequencing requirements must be followed if multiple coding is indicated for any diagnoses. If a V-code is reported in place of a case mix diagnosis, then optional item M1024 **Payment Diagnoses** (Columns 3 and 4) may be completed. A case mix diagnosis is a diagnosis that determines the Medicare PPS case mix group. Do not assign symptom control ratings for V- or E-codes.

Code each row according to the following directions for each column:

Column 1: Enter the description of the diagnosis.
Column 2: Enter the ICD-10CM code for the diagnosis described in Column 1.

Rate the degree of symptom control for the condition listed in Column 1 using the following scale:
0 - Asymptomatic, no treatment needed at this time
1 - Symptoms well controlled with current therapy

2 - Symptoms controlled with difficulty, affecting daily functioning; patient needs ongoing monitoring
3 - Symptoms poorly controlled; patient needs frequent adjustment in treatment and dose monitoring
4 - Symptoms poorly controlled; history of re-hospitalizations

Note that in Column 2 the rating for symptom control of each diagnosis should not be used to determine the sequencing of the diagnoses listed in Column 1. These are separate items and sequencing may not coincide. Sequencing of diagnoses should reflect the seriousness of each condition and support the disciplines and services provided.

Column 3: (OPTIONAL) If a V-code is assigned to any row in Column 2, in place of a case mix diagnosis, it may be necessary to complete optional item M1024 **Payment Diagnoses** (Columns 3 and 4). See OASIS-C Guidance Manual.

Column 4: (OPTIONAL) If a V-code in Column 2 is reported in place of a case mix diagnosis that requires multiple diagnosis codes under ICD-10-CM coding guidelines, enter the diagnosis descriptions and the ICD-10-CM codes in the same row in Columns 3 and 4. For example, if the case mix diagnosis is a manifestation code, record the diagnosis description and ICD-10-CM code for the underlying condition in Column 3 of that row and the diagnosis description and ICD-10-CM code for the manifestation in Column 4 of that row. Otherwise, leave Column 4 blank in that row.

(M1020) Primary Diagnosis and (M1022) Other Diagnoses			(M1024) Payment Diagnoses (OPTIONAL)	
Column 1	Column 2	Column 3		Column 4
Diagnoses (Sequencing of diagnoses should reflect the seriousness of each condition and support the disciplines and services provided.)	ICD-10-CM and symptom control rating for each condition. Note that the sequencing of these ratings may not match the sequencing of the diagnoses	Complete if a V-code is assigned under certain circumstances to Column 2 in place of a case mix diagnosis.		Complete **only if** the V-code in Column 2 is reported in place of a case mix diagnosis that is a multiple coding situation (e.g., a manifestation code).
Description	ICD-10-CM / Symptom Control Rating	Description/ ICD-10-CM		Description/ ICD-10-CM
(M1020) Primary Diagnosis a. _____	(V-codes are allowed) a. (___.___) ☐0 ☐1 ☐2 ☐3 ☐4	(V- or E-codes NOT allowed) a. (___.___)		(V- or E-codes NOT allowed) a. (___.___)
(M1022) Other Diagnoses b. _____	(V- or E-codes are allowed) b. (___.___) ☐0 ☐1 ☐2 ☐3 ☐4	(V- or E-codes NOT allowed) b. (___.___)		(V- or E-codes NOT allowed) b. (___.___)

(continued)

(M1020) Primary Diagnosis and (M1022) Other Diagnoses

(M1024) Payment Diagnoses (OPTIONAL)

Column 1	Column 2	Column 3	Column 4
c. _____	c. (___ ___ . ___ ___) ☐0 ☐1 ☐2 ☐3 ☐4	c. (___ ___ ___ . ___ ___)	c. (___ ___ ___ . ___ ___)
d. _____	d. (___ ___ . ___ ___) ☐0 ☐1 ☐2 ☐3 ☐4	d. (___ ___ ___ . ___ ___)	d. (___ ___ ___ . ___ ___)
e. _____	e. (___ ___ . ___ ___) ☐0 ☐1 ☐2 ☐3 ☐4	e. (___ ___ ___ . ___ ___)	e. (___ ___ ___ . ___ ___)
f. _____	f. (___ ___ . ___ ___) ☐0 ☐1 ☐2 ☐3 ☐4	f. (___ ___ ___ . ___ ___)	f. (___ ___ ___ . ___ ___)

(M1030) **Therapies** the patient receives at home: **(Mark all that apply.)**

- ☐ 1 - Intravenous or infusion therapy (excludes TPN [total parenteral nutrition])
- ☐ 2 - Parenteral nutrition (TPN or lipids)
- ☐ 3 - Enteral nutrition (nasogastric, gastrostomy, jejunostomy, or any other artificial entry into the alimentary canal)
- ☐ 4 - None of the above

(M1032) **Risk for Hospitalization:** Which of the following signs or symptoms characterize this patient as at risk for hospitalization? **(Mark all that apply.)**

- ☐ 1 - Recent decline in mental, emotional, or behavioral status
- ☐ 2 - Multiple hospitalizations (two or more) in the past 12 months
- ☐ 3 - History of falls (two or more falls—or any fall with an injury—in the past year)
- ☐ 4 - Taking five or more medications
- ☐ 5 - Frailty indicators, for example, weight loss, self-reported exhaustion
- ☐ 6 - Other
- ☐ 7 - None of the above

(M1034) **Overall Status:** Which description best fits the patient's overall status? **(Check one.)**

- ☐ 0 - The patient is stable with no heightened risk(s) for serious complications and death (beyond those typical of the patient's age).
- ☐ 1 - The patient is temporarily facing high health risk(s) but is likely to return to being stable without heightened risk(s) for serious complications and death (beyond those typical of the patient's age).

☐ 2 - The patient is likely to remain in fragile health and have ongoing high risk(s) of serious complications and death.
☐ 3 - The patient has serious progressive conditions that could lead to death within a year.
☐ UK - The patient's situation is unknown or unclear.

(M1036) **Risk Factors**, either present or past, likely to affect current health status and/or outcome: **(Mark all that apply.)**

☐ 1 - Smoking
☐ 2 - Obesity
☐ 3 - Alcohol dependency
☐ 4 - Drug dependency
☐ 5 - None of the above
☐ UK - Unknown

(M1040) **Influenza Vaccine:** Did the patient receive the influenza vaccine from your agency for this year's influenza season (October 1 through March 31) during this episode of care?

☐ 0 - No
☐ 1 - Yes [*Go to M1050*]
☐ NA - Does not apply because entire episode of care (SOC/ROC to Transfer/Discharge) is outside this influenza season. [*Go to M1050*]

(M1045) **Reason Influenza Vaccine Not Received:** If the patient did not receive the influenza vaccine from your agency during this episode of care, state reason.

☐ 1 - Received from another health care provider (e.g., physician)
☐ 2 - Received from your agency previously during this year's flu season
☐ 3 - Offered and declined

☐ 4 - Assessed and determined to have medical contraindication(s)
☐ 5 - Not indicated; patient does not meet age/condition guidelines for influenza vaccine
☐ 6 - Inability to obtain vaccine due to declared shortage
☐ 7 - None of the above

(M1050) **Pneumococcal Vaccine:** Did the patient receive pneumococcal polysaccharide vaccine (PPV) from your agency during this episode of care (SOC/ROC to Transfer [TRN]/Discharge [DC])?

☐ 0 - No
☐ 1 - Yes [*Go to M1500 at TRN; Go to M1230 at DC*]

(M1055) **Reason PPV Not Received:** If patient did not receive the pneumococcal polysaccharide vaccine (PPV) from your agency during this episode of care (SOC/ROC to Transfer/Discharge), state reason:

☐ 1 - Patient has received PPV in the past
☐ 2 - Offered and declined
☐ 3 - Assessed and determined to have medical contraindication(s)
☐ 4 - Not indicated; patient does not meet age/condition guidelines for PPV
☐ 5 - None of the above

LIVING ARRANGEMENTS

(M1100) **Patient Living Situation:** Which of the following best describes the patient's residential circumstance and availability of assistance? **(Check one box only.)**

Living Arrangement	Availability of Assistance				
	Around the clock	Regular daytime	Regular nighttime	Occasional/ short-term assistance	No assistance available
a. Patient lives alone	☐ 01	☐ 02	☐ 03	☐ 04	☐ 05
b. Patient lives with other person(s) in the home	☐ 06	☐ 07	☐ 08	☐ 09	☐ 10
c. Patient lives in congregate situation (e.g., assisted living)	☐ 11	☐ 12	☐ 13	☐ 14	☐ 15

SENSORY STATUS

(M1200) **Vision** (with corrective lenses if the patient usually wears them):

☐ 0 - Normal Vision: sees adequately in most situations; can see medication labels, newsprint.

☐ 1 - Partially Impaired: cannot see medication labels or newsprint, but can see obstacles in path, and the surrounding layout; can count fingers at arm's length.

☐ 2 - Severely Impaired: cannot locate objects without hearing or touching them or patient nonresponsive.

(M1210) **Ability to hear** (with hearing aid or hearing appliance if normally used):

- ☐ 0 - Adequate: hears normal conversation without difficulty.
- ☐ 1 - Mildly to Moderately Impaired: difficulty hearing in some environments or speaker may need to increase volume or speak distinctly.
- ☐ 2 - Severely Impaired: absence of useful hearing.
- ☐ UK - Unable to assess hearing.

(M1220) **Understanding of Verbal Content** in patient's own language (with hearing aid or device if used):

- ☐ 0 - Understands: clear comprehension without cues or repetitions.
- ☐ 1 - Usually Understands: understands most conversations, but misses some part/intent of message. Requires cues at times to understand.
- ☐ 2 - Sometimes Understands: understands only basic conversations or simple, direct phrases. Frequently requires cues to understand.
- ☐ 3 - Rarely/Never Understands
- ☐ UK - Unable to assess understanding.

(M1230) **Speech and Oral (Verbal) Expression of Language (in Patient's Own Language)**:

- ☐ 0 - Expresses complex ideas, feelings, and needs clearly, completely, and easily in all situations with no observable impairment.
- ☐ 1 - Minimal difficulty in expressing ideas and needs (may take extra time; makes occasional errors in word choice, grammar or speech intelligibility; needs minimal prompting or assistance).
- ☐ 2 - Expresses simple ideas or needs with moderate difficulty (needs prompting or assistance, errors

in word choice, organization or speech intelligibility). Speaks in phrases or short sentences.
- ☐ 3 - Has severe difficulty expressing basic ideas or needs and requires maximal assistance or guessing by listener. Speech limited to single words or short phrases.
- ☐ 4 - Unable to express basic needs even with maximal prompting or assistance but is not comatose or unresponsive (e.g., speech is nonsensical or unintelligible).
- ☐ 5 - Patient nonresponsive or unable to speak.

(M1240) Has this patient had a formal **Pain Assessment** using a standardized pain assessment tool (appropriate to the patient's ability to communicate the severity of pain)?

- ☐ 0 - No standardized assessment conducted
- ☐ 1 - Yes, and it does not indicate severe pain
- ☐ 2 - Yes, and it indicates severe pain

(M1242) **Frequency of Pain Interfering** with patient's activity or movement:

- ☐ 0 - Patient has no pain
- ☐ 1 - Patient has pain that does not interfere with activity or movement
- ☐ 2 - Less often than daily
- ☐ 3 - Daily, but not constantly
- ☐ 4 - All of the time

INTEGUMENTARY STATUS

(M1300) **Pressure Ulcer Assessment:** Was this patient assessed for **Risk of Developing Pressure Ulcers**?

- ☐ 0 - No assessment conducted [*Go to M1306*]

☐ 1 - Yes, based on an evaluation of clinical factors, for example, mobility, incontinence, nutrition, etc., without use of standardized tool
☐ 2 - Yes, using a standardized tool, for example, Braden, Norton, other

(M1302) Does this patient have a **Risk of Developing Pressure Ulcers?**

☐ 0 - No
☐ 1 - Yes

(M1306) Does this patient have at least one **Unhealed Pressure Ulcer at Stage II or Higher** or designated as "unstageable"?

☐ 0 - No [*Go to M1322*]
☐ 1 - Yes

(M1307) **The Oldest Nonepithelialized Stage II Pressure Ulcer That Is Present at Discharge**

☐ 1 - Was present at the most recent SOC/ROC assessment
☐ 2 - Developed since the most recent SOC/ROC assessment: record date pressure ulcer first identified:
__ __ / __ __ / __ __
month / day / year
☐ NA - No nonepithelialized Stage II pressure ulcers are present at discharge

(M1308) **Current Number of Unhealed (Nonepithelialized) Pressure Ulcers at Each Stage:** (Enter "0" if none; excludes Stage I pressure ulcers)

	Column 1 Complete at SOC/ROC/FU and DC	Column 2 Complete at FU and DC
Stage description – unhealed pressure ulcers	Number currently present	Number of those listed in Column 1 that were present on admission (most recent SOC/ROC)
a. **Stage II:** Partial thickness loss of dermis presenting as a shallow open ulcer with red pink wound bed, without slough. May also present as an intact or open/ruptured serum-filled blister.	_____	_____
b. **Stage III:** Full thickness tissue loss. Subcutaneous fat may be visible but bone, tendon, or muscles are not exposed. Slough may be present but does not obscure the depth of tissue loss. May include undermining and tunneling.	_____	_____
c. **Stage IV:** Full thickness tissue loss with visible bone, tendon, or muscle. Slough or eschar may be present on some parts of the wound bed. Often includes undermining and tunneling.	_____	_____
d.1 Unstageable: Known or likely but unstageable due to non-removable dressing or device	_____	_____

	Column 1 Complete at SOC/ROC/FU and DC	Column 2 Complete at FU and DC
Stage description – unhealed pressure ulcers	Number currently present	Number of those listed in Column 1 that were present on admission (most recent SOC/ROC)
d.2 Unstageable: Known or likely but unstageable due to coverage of wound bed by slough and/or eschar.	_____	_____
d.3 Unstageable: Suspected deep tissue injury in evolution.	_____	_____

DC, discharge; FU, follow-up; ROC, resumption of care; SOC, start of care.

Directions for M1310, M1312, and M1314: If the patient has one or more unhealed (nonepithelialized) Stage III or IV pressure ulcers, identify the **Stage III or IV pressure ulcer with the largest surface dimension (length × width)** and record in centimeters. If no Stage III or Stage IV pressure ulcers, go to M1320.

(M1310) **Pressure Ulcer Length:** Longest length "head-to-toe"
| ___ | ___ | . | ___ | (cm)

(M1312) **Pressure Ulcer Width:** Width of the same pressure ulcer; greatest width perpendicular to the length
| ___ | ___ | . | ___ | (cm)

(M1314) **Pressure Ulcer Depth:** Depth of the same pressure ulcer; from visible surface to the deepest area
| ___ | ___ | . | ___ | (cm)

(M1320) **Status of Most Problematic (Observable) Pressure Ulcer:**
- ☐ 0 - Newly epithelialized
- ☐ 1 - Fully granulating
- ☐ 2 - Early/partial granulation
- ☐ 3 - Not healing
- ☐ NA - No observable pressure ulcer

(M1322) **Current Number of Stage I Pressure Ulcers:** Intact skin with nonblanchable redness of a localized area usually over a bony prominence. The area may be painful, firm, soft, warmer or cooler as compared to adjacent tissue.

☐ 0   ☐ 1   ☐ 2   ☐ 3   ☐ 4 or more

(M1324) **Stage of Most Problematic Unhealed (Observable) Pressure Ulcer:**
- ☐ 1 - Stage I
- ☐ 2 - Stage II
- ☐ 3 - Stage III
- ☐ 4 - Stage IV
- ☐ NA - No observable pressure ulcer or unhealed pressure ulcer

(M1330) Does this patient have a **Stasis Ulcer**?
- ☐ 0 - No [*Go to M1340*]
- ☐ 1 - Yes, patient has BOTH observable and unobservable stasis ulcers
- ☐ 2 - Yes, patient has observable stasis ulcers ONLY
- ☐ 3 - Yes, patient has unobservable stasis ulcers ONLY (known but not observable due to nonremovable dressing) [*Go to M1340*]

(M1332) Current Number of (Observable) Stasis Ulcer(s):

☐ 1 - One
☐ 2 - Two
☐ 3 - Three
☐ 4 - Four or more

(M1334) Status of Most Problematic (Observable) Stasis Ulcer:

☐ 0 - Newly epithelialized
☐ 1 - Fully granulating
☐ 2 - Early/partial granulation
☐ 3 - Not healing

(M1340) Does this patient have a **Surgical Wound?**

☐ 0 - No [*Go to M1350*]
☐ 1 - Yes, patient has at least one (observable) surgical wound
☐ 2 - Surgical wound known but not observable due to nonremovable dressing [*Go to M1350*]

(M1342) Status of Most Problematic (Observable) Surgical Wound:

☐ 0 - Newly epithelialized
☐ 1 - Fully granulating
☐ 2 - Early/partial granulation
☐ 3 - Not healing

(M1350) Does this patient have a **Skin Lesion** or **Open Wound**, excluding bowel ostomy, other than those described above *that is receiving intervention* by the home health agency?

☐ 0 - No
☐ 1 - Yes

RESPIRATORY STATUS

(M1400) When is the patient dyspneic or noticeably **Short of Breath?**

- ☐ 0 - Patient is not short of breath
- ☐ 1 - When walking more than 20 feet, climbing stairs
- ☐ 2 - With moderate exertion (e.g., while dressing, using commode or bedpan, walking distances less than 20 feet)
- ☐ 3 - With minimal exertion (e.g., while eating, talking, or performing other activities of daily living [ADL] or with agitation
- ☐ 4 - At rest (during day or night)

(M1410) **Respiratory Treatments** utilized at home: **(Mark all that apply.)**

- ☐ 1 - Oxygen (intermittent or continuous)
- ☐ 2 - Ventilator (continually or at night)
- ☐ 3 - Continuous/bi-level positive airway pressure
- ☐ 4 - None of the above

CARDIAC STATUS

(M1500) **Symptoms in Heart Failure Patients**: If patient has been diagnosed with heart failure, did the patient exhibit symptoms indicated by clinical heart failure guidelines (including dyspnea, orthopnea, edema, or weight gain) at any point since the previous OASIS assessment?

- ☐ 0 - No [*Go to M2004 at TRN; Go to M1600 at DC*]
- ☐ 1 - Yes
- ☐ 2 - Not assessed [*Go to M2004 at TRN; Go to M1600 at DC*]
- ☐ NA - Patient does not have diagnosis of heart failure [*Go to M2004 at TRN; Go to M1600 at DC*]

(M1510) **Heart Failure Follow-Up:** If patient has been diagnosed with heart failure and has exhibited symptoms indicative of heart failure since the previous OASIS assessment, what action(s) has (have) been taken to respond? **(Mark all that apply.)**

☐ 0 - No action taken
☐ 1 - Patient's physician (or other primary care practitioner) contacted the same day
☐ 2 - Patient advised to get emergency treatment (e.g., call 911 or go to emergency department)
☐ 3 - Implemented physician-ordered patient-specific established parameters for treatment
☐ 4 - Patient education or other clinical interventions
☐ 5 - Obtained change in care plan orders (e.g., increased monitoring by agency, change in visit frequency, telehealth, etc.)

ELIMINATION STATUS

(M1600) Has this patient been treated for a **Urinary Tract Infection** in the past 14 days?

☐ 0 - No
☐ 1 - Yes
☐ NA - Patient on prophylactic treatment
☐ UK - Unknown **[Omit "UK" option on DC]**

(M1610) **Urinary Incontinence or Urinary Catheter Presence:**

☐ 0 - No incontinence or catheter (includes anuria or ostomy for urinary drainage) [*Go to M1620*]
☐ 1 - Patient is incontinent
☐ 2 - Patient requires a urinary catheter (i.e., external, indwelling, intermittent, suprapubic) [*Go to M1620*]

(M1615) When does **Urinary Incontinence** occur?

☐ 0 - Timed-voiding defers incontinence
☐ 1 - Occasional stress incontinence
☐ 2 - During the night only
☐ 3 - During the day only
☐ 4 - During the day and night

(M1620) **Bowel Incontinence Frequency:**

☐ 0 - Very rarely or never has bowel incontinence
☐ 1 - Less than once weekly
☐ 2 - One to three times weekly
☐ 3 - Four to six times weekly
☐ 4 - On a daily basis
☐ 5 - More often than once daily
☐ NA - Patient has ostomy for bowel elimination
☐ UK - Unknown **[Omit "UK" option on FU, DC]**

(M1630) **Ostomy for Bowel Elimination:** Does this patient have an ostomy for bowel elimination that (within the past 14 days): (a) was related to an inpatient facility stay, *or* (b) necessitated a change in medical or treatment regimen?

☐ 0 - Patient does *not* have an ostomy for bowel elimination.
☐ 1 - Patient's ostomy was *not* related to an inpatient stay and did *not* necessitate change in medical or treatment regimen.
☐ 2 - The ostomy *was* related to an inpatient stay or *did* necessitate change in medical or treatment regimen.

NEURO/EMOTIONAL/BEHAVIORAL STATUS

(M1700) **Cognitive Functioning:** Patient's current (day of assessment) level of alertness, orientation, comprehension, concentration, and immediate memory for simple commands.

- ☐ 0 - Alert/oriented, able to focus and shift attention, comprehends and recalls task directions independently.
- ☐ 1 - Requires prompting (cuing, repetition, reminders) only under stressful or unfamiliar conditions.
- ☐ 2 - Requires assistance and some direction in specific situations (e.g., on all tasks involving shifting of attention), or consistently requires low stimulus environment due to distractibility.
- ☐ 3 - Requires considerable assistance in routine situations. Is not alert and oriented or is unable to shift attention and recall directions more than half the time.
- ☐ 4 - Totally dependent due to disturbances such as constant disorientation, coma, persistent vegetative state, or delirium.

(M1710) When Confused (Reported or Observed Within the Past 14 Days):

- ☐ 0 - Never
- ☐ 1 - In new or complex situations only
- ☐ 2 - On awakening or at night only
- ☐ 3 - During the day and evening, but not constantly
- ☐ 4 - Constantly
- ☐ NA - Patient nonresponsive

(M1720) When Anxious (Reported or Observed Within the Past 14 Days):

- ☐ 0 - None of the time
- ☐ 1 - Less often than daily
- ☐ 2 - Daily, but not constantly

☐ 3 - All of the time
☐ NA - Patient nonresponsive

(M1730) **Depression Screening:** Has the patient been screened for depression, using a standardized depression screening tool?

☐ 0 - No
☐ 1 - Yes, patient was screened using the PHQ-2©* scale. (Instructions for this two-question tool: Ask patient: "Over the past 2 weeks, how often have you been bothered by any of the following problems?")

PHQ-2©*	Not at all (0–1 day)	Several days (2–6 days)	More than half of the days (7–11 days)	Nearly every day (12–14 days)	N/A Unable to respond
a. Little interest or pleasure in doing things?	☐ 0	☐ 1	☐ 2	☐ 3	☐ na
b. Feeling down, depressed, or hopeless?	☐ 0	☐ 1	☐ 2	☐ 3	☐ na

☐ 2 - Yes, with a different standardized assessment—and the patient meets criteria for further evaluation for depression.
☐ 3 - Yes, patient was screened with a different standardized assessment—and the patient does not meet criteria for further evaluation for depression.

Copyright© Pfizer Inc. All rights reserved. Reproduced with permission.

(M1740) **Cognitive, behavioral, and psychiatric symptoms** that are demonstrated at least once a week (**Reported or Observed**): **(Mark all that apply.)**

- ☐ 1 - Memory deficit: failure to recognize familiar persons/places, inability to recall events of past 24 hours, significant memory loss so that supervision is required
- ☐ 2 - Impaired decision making: failure to perform usual ADL or instrumental activities of daily living (IADL), inability to appropriately stop activities, jeopardizes safety through actions
- ☐ 3 - Verbal disruption: yelling, threatening, excessive profanity, sexual references, etc.
- ☐ 4 - Physical aggression: aggressive or combative to self and others (e.g., hits self, throws objects, punches, dangerous maneuvers with wheelchair or other objects)
- ☐ 5 - Disruptive, infantile, or socially inappropriate behavior (**excludes** verbal actions)
- ☐ 6 - Delusional, hallucinatory, or paranoid behavior
- ☐ 7 - None of the above behaviors demonstrated

(M1745) **Frequency of Disruptive Behavior Symptoms (Reported or Observed)** Any physical, verbal, or other disruptive/dangerous symptoms that are injurious to self or others or jeopardize personal safety.

- ☐ 0 - Never
- ☐ 1 - Less than once a month
- ☐ 2 - Once a month
- ☐ 3 - Several times each month
- ☐ 4 - Several times a week
- ☐ 5 - At least daily

(M1750) Is this patient receiving **Psychiatric Nursing Services** at home provided by a qualified psychiatric nurse?

☐ 0 - No
☐ 1 - Yes

ADL/IADL

(M1800) **Grooming:** Current ability to tend safely to personal hygiene needs (i.e., washing face and hands, hair care, shaving or makeup, teeth or denture care, fingernail care).

☐ 0 - Able to groom self unaided, with or without the use of assistive devices or adapted methods.
☐ 1 - Grooming utensils must be placed within reach before able to complete grooming activities.
☐ 2 - Someone must assist the patient to groom self.
☐ 3 - Patient depends entirely upon someone else for grooming needs.

(M1810) Current **Ability to Dress Upper Body** safely (with or without dressing aids) including undergarments, pullovers, front-opening shirts and blouses, managing zippers, buttons, and snaps:

☐ 0 - Able to get clothes out of closets and drawers, put them on and remove them from the upper body without assistance.
☐ 1 - Able to dress upper body without assistance if clothing is laid out or handed to the patient.
☐ 2 - Someone must help the patient put on upper body clothing.
☐ 3 - Patient depends entirely upon another person to dress the upper body.

(M1820) Current **Ability to Dress Lower Body** safely (with or without dressing aids) including undergarments, slacks, socks or nylons, shoes:

☐ 0 - Able to obtain, put on, and remove clothing and shoes without assistance.
☐ 1 - Able to dress lower body without assistance if clothing and shoes are laid out or handed to the patient.
☐ 2 - Someone must help the patient put on undergarments, slacks, socks or nylons, and shoes.
☐ 3 - Patient depends entirely upon another person to dress lower body.

(M1830) **Bathing:** Current ability to wash entire body safely. **Excludes grooming (washing face, washing hands, and shampooing hair).**
☐ 0 - Able to bathe self in shower or tub independently, including getting in and out of tub/shower.
☐ 1 - With the use of devices, is able to bathe self in shower or tub independently, including getting in and out of the tub/shower.
☐ 2 - Able to bathe in shower or tub with the intermittent assistance of another person:
   (a) for intermittent supervision or encouragement or reminders, OR
   (b) to get in and out of the shower or tub, OR
   (c) for washing difficult to reach areas.
☐ 3 - Able to participate in bathing self in shower or tub, but requires presence of another person throughout the bath for assistance or supervision.
☐ 4 - Unable to use the shower or tub, but able to bathe self independently with or without the use of devices at the sink, in chair, or on commode.

☐ 5 - Unable to use the shower or tub, but able to participate in bathing self in bed, at the sink, in bedside chair, or on commode, with the assistance or supervision of another person throughout the bath.
☐ 6 - Unable to participate effectively in bathing and is bathed totally by another person.

(M1840) **Toilet Transferring:** Current ability to get to and from the toilet or bedside commode safely and transfer on and off toilet/commode.

☐ 0 - Able to get to and from the toilet and transfer independently with or without a device.
☐ 1 - When reminded, assisted, or supervised by another person, able to get to and from the toilet and transfer.
☐ 2 - *Unable* to get to and from the toilet but is able to use a bedside commode (with or without assistance).
☐ 3 - *Unable* to get to and from the toilet or bedside commode but is able to use a bedpan/urinal independently.
☐ 4 - Is totally dependent in toileting.

(M1845) **Toileting Hygiene:** Current ability to maintain perineal hygiene safely, adjust clothes and/or incontinence pads before and after using toilet, commode, bedpan, urinal. If managing ostomy, includes cleaning area around stoma, but not managing equipment.

☐ 0 - Able to manage toileting hygiene and clothing management without assistance.
☐ 1 - Able to manage toileting hygiene and clothing management without assistance if supplies/implements are laid out for the patient.

- ☐ 2 - Someone must help the patient to maintain toileting hygiene and/or adjust clothing.
- ☐ 3 - Patient depends entirely upon another person to maintain toileting hygiene.

(M1850) **Transferring:** Current ability to move safely from bed to chair, or ability to turn and position self in bed if patient is bedfast.

- ☐ 0 - Able to independently transfer.
- ☐ 1 - Able to transfer with minimal human assistance or with use of an assistive device.
- ☐ 2 - Able to bear weight and pivot during the transfer process but unable to transfer self.
- ☐ 3 - Unable to transfer self and is unable to bear weight or pivot when transferred by another person.
- ☐ 4 - Bedfast, unable to transfer but is able to turn and position self in bed.
- ☐ 5 - Bedfast, unable to transfer and is unable to turn and position self.

(M1860) **Ambulation/Locomotion:** Current ability to walk safely, once in a standing position, or use a wheelchair, once in a seated position, on a variety of surfaces.

- ☐ 0 - Able to independently walk on even and uneven surfaces and negotiate stairs with or without railings (i.e., needs no human assistance or assistive device).
- ☐ 1 - With the use of a one-handed device (e.g., cane, single crutch, hemi-walker), able to independently walk on even and uneven surfaces and negotiate stairs with or without railings.
- ☐ 2 - Requires use of a two-handed device (e.g., walker or crutches) to walk alone on a level surface and/or requires human supervision or assistance to negotiate stairs or steps or uneven surfaces.

- ☐ 3 - Able to walk only with the supervision or assistance of another person at all times.
- ☐ 4 - Chairfast, *unable* to ambulate but is able to wheel self independently.
- ☐ 5 - Chairfast, unable to ambulate and is *unable* to wheel self.
- ☐ 6 - Bedfast, unable to ambulate or be up in a chair.

(M1870) **Feeding or Eating:** Current ability to feed self meals and snacks safely. Note: This refers only to the process of *eating, chewing,* and *swallowing, not preparing* the food to be eaten.

- ☐ 0 - Able to independently feed self.
- ☐ 1 - Able to feed self independently but requires:
    (a) meal set-up; OR
    (b) intermittent assistance or supervision from another person; OR
    (c) a liquid, pureed, or ground meat diet.
- ☐ 2 - *Unable* to feed self and must be assisted or supervised throughout the meal/snack.
- ☐ 3 - Able to take in nutrients orally *and* receive supplemental nutrients through a nasogastric tube or gastrostomy.
- ☐ 4 - *Unable* to take in nutrients orally and is fed nutrients through a nasogastric tube or gastrostomy.
- ☐ 5 - Unable to take in nutrients orally or by tube feeding.

(M1880) Current **Ability to Plan and Prepare Light Meals** (e.g., cereal, sandwich) or reheat delivered meals safely:

- ☐ 0 - (a) Able to independently plan and prepare all light meals for self or reheat delivered meals; OR

(b) Is physically, cognitively, and mentally able to prepare light meals on a regular basis but has not routinely performed light meal preparation in the past (i.e., prior to this home care admission).
☐ 1 - *Unable* to prepare light meals on a regular basis due to physical, cognitive, or mental limitations.
☐ 2 - Unable to prepare any light meals or reheat any delivered meals.

(M1890) **Ability to Use Telephone:** Current ability to answer the phone safely, including dialing numbers, and *effectively* using the telephone to communicate.
☐ 0 - Able to dial numbers and answer calls appropriately and as desired.
☐ 1 - Able to use a specially adapted telephone (i.e., large numbers on the dial, teletype phone for the deaf) and call essential numbers.
☐ 2 - Able to answer the telephone and carry on a normal conversation but has difficulty with placing calls.
☐ 3 - Able to answer the telephone only some of the time or is able to carry on only a limited conversation.
☐ 4 - *Unable* to answer the telephone at all but can listen if assisted with equipment.
☐ 5 - Totally unable to use the telephone.
☐ NA - Patient does not have a telephone.

(M1900) **Prior Functioning ADL/IADL:** Indicate the patient's usual ability with everyday activities prior to this current illness, exacerbation, or injury. Check only *one* box in each row.

Functional Area	Independent	Needed Some Help	Dependent
a. Self-care (e.g., grooming, dressing, and bathing)	☐ 0	☐ 1	☐ 2
b. Ambulation	☐ 0	☐ 1	☐ 2
c. Transfer	☐ 0	☐ 1	☐ 2
d. Household tasks (e.g., light meal preparation, laundry, shopping)	☐ 0	☐ 1	☐ 2

(M1910) Has this patient had a multi-factor **Fall Risk Assessment** (such as falls history, use of multiple medications, mental impairment, toileting frequency, general mobility/transferring impairment, environmental hazards)?
 ☐ 0 - No multi-factor falls risk assessment conducted.
 ☐ 1 - Yes, and it does not indicate a risk for falls.
 ☐ 2 - Yes, and it indicates a risk for falls.

MEDICATIONS

(M2000) **Drug Regimen Review:** Does a complete drug regimen review indicate potential clinically significant medication issues, for example, drug reactions, ineffective drug therapy, side effects, drug interactions, duplicate therapy, omissions, dosage errors, or noncompliance?
 ☐ 0 - Not assessed/reviewed [*Go to M2010*]
 ☐ 1 - No problems found during review [*Go to M2010*]
 ☐ 2 - Problems found during review
 ☐ NA - Patient is not taking any medications [*Go to M2040*]

(M2002) **Medication Follow-Up:** Was a physician or the physician-designee contacted within one calendar day to resolve clinically significant medication issues, including reconciliation?

- ☐ 0 - No
- ☐ 1 - Yes

(M2004) **Medication Intervention:** If there were any clinically significant medication issues since the previous OASIS assessment, was a physician or the physician-designee contacted within 1 calendar day of the assessment to resolve clinically significant medication issues, including reconciliation?

- ☐ 0 - No
- ☐ 1 - Yes
- ☐ NA - No clinically significant medication issues identified since the previous OASIS assessment

(M2010) **Patient/Caregiver High-Risk Drug Education:** Has the patient/caregiver received instruction on special precautions for all high-risk medications (such as hypoglycemics, anticoagulants, etc.) and how and when to report problems that may occur?

- ☐ 0 - No
- ☐ 1 - Yes
- ☐ NA - Patient not taking any high-risk drugs OR patient/caregiver fully knowledgeable about special precautions associated with all high-risk medications

(M2015) **Patient/Caregiver Drug Education Intervention:** Since the previous OASIS assessment, was the patient/

caregiver instructed by agency staff or other health care provider to monitor the effectiveness of drug therapy, drug reactions, and side effects, and how and when to report problems that may occur?

☐ 0 - No
☐ 1 - Yes
☐ NA - Patient not taking any drugs

(M2020) **Management of Oral Medications:** *Patient's current ability* to prepare and take *all* oral medications reliably and safely, including administration of the correct dosage at the appropriate times/intervals. *Excludes* **injectable and IV medications. (NOTE: This refers to ability, not compliance or willingness.)**

☐ 0 - Able to independently take the correct oral medication(s) and proper dosage(s) at the correct times.
☐ 1 - Able to take medication(s) at the correct times if:
  (a) individual dosages are prepared in advance by another person; OR
  (b) another person develops a drug diary or chart.
☐ 2 - Able to take medication(s) at the correct times if given reminders by another person at the appropriate times
☐ 3 - *Unable* to take medication unless administered by another person.
☐ NA - No oral medications prescribed.

(M2030) **Management of Injectable Medications:** *Patient's current ability* to prepare and take *all* prescribed injectable medications reliably and safely, including administration of correct dosage at the appropriate times/intervals. *Excludes* **IV medications.**

☐ 0 - Able to independently take the correct medication(s) and proper dosage(s) at the correct times.
☐ 1 - Able to take injectable medication(s) at the correct times if:
(a) individual syringes are prepared in advance by another person; OR
(b) another person develops a drug diary or chart.
☐ 2 - Able to take medication(s) at the correct times if given reminders by another person based on the frequency of the injection
☐ 3 - *Unable* to take injectable medication unless administered by another person.
☐ NA - No injectable medications prescribed.

(M2040) **Prior Medication Management:** Indicate the patient's usual ability with managing oral and injectable medications prior to this current illness, exacerbation, or injury. Check only **one** box in each row.

Functional Area	Independent	Needed Some Help	Dependent	Not Applicable
a. Oral medications	☐ 0	☐ 1	☐ 2	☐ na
b. Injectable medications	☐ 0	☐ 1	☐ 2	☐ na

CARE MANAGEMENT

(M2100) **Types and Sources of Assistance:** Determine the level of caregiver ability and willingness to provide assistance for the following activities, if assistance is needed. (Check only *one* box in each row.)

Type of Assistance	No assistance needed in this area	Caregiver(s) currently provide assistance	Caregiver(s) need training/supportive services to provide assistance	Caregiver(s) not likely to provide assistance	Unclear if Caregiver(s) will provide assistance	Assistance needed, but no Caregiver(s) available
a. **ADL assistance** (e.g., transfer/ambulation, bathing, dressing, toileting, eating/feeding)	☐ 0	☐ 1	☐ 2	☐ 3	☐ 4	☐ 5
b. **IADL assistance** (e.g., meals, housekeeping, laundry, telephone, shopping, finances)	☐ 0	☐ 1	☐ 2	☐ 3	☐ 4	☐ 5
c. **Medication administration** (e.g., oral, inhaled, or injectable)	☐ 0	☐ 1	☐ 2	☐ 3	☐ 4	☐ 5
d. **Medical procedures/treatments** (e.g., changing wound dressing)	☐ 0	☐ 1	☐ 2	☐ 3	☐ 4	☐ 5

7. HOME HEALTH SERVICES   171

Type of Assistance	No assistance needed in this area	Caregiver(s) currently provide assistance	Caregiver(s) need training/ supportive services to provide assistance	Caregiver(s) not likely to provide assistance	Unclear if Caregiver(s) will provide assistance	Assistance needed, but no Caregiver(s) available
e. **Management of equipment** (includes oxygen, IV/infusion equipment, enteral/parenteral nutrition, ventilator therapy equipment or supplies)	☐ 0	☐ 1	☐ 2	☐ 3	☐ 4	☐ 5
f. **Supervision and safety** (e.g., due to cognitive impairment)	☐ 0	☐ 1	☐ 2	☐ 3	☐ 4	☐ 5
g. **Advocacy or facilitation** of patient's participation in appropriate medical care (includes transportation to or from appointments)	☐ 0	☐ 1	☐ 2	☐ 3	☐ 4	☐ 5

(M2110) How Often does the patient receive **ADL or IADL assistance** from any caregiver(s) (other than home health agency staff)?

- ☐ 1 - At least daily
- ☐ 2 - Three or more times per week
- ☐ 3 - One to two times per week
- ☐ 4 - Received, but less often than weekly
- ☐ 5 - No assistance received
- ☐ UK - Unknown **[Omit "UK" option on DC]**

THERAPY NEED AND PLAN OF CARE

(M2200) **Therapy Need:** In the home health plan of care for the Medicare payment episode for which this assessment will define a case mix group, what is the indicated need for therapy visits (total of reasonable and necessary physical, occupational, and speech-language pathology visits combined)? **(Enter zero ["000"] if no therapy visits indicated.)**

(__ __ __) Number of therapy visits indicated (total of physical, occupational, and speech-language pathology combined).

☐ NA - Not Applicable: No case mix group defined by this assessment.

(M2250) **Plan of Care Synopsis:** (Check only *one* box in each row.) Does the physician-ordered plan of care include the following:

Plan/Intervention	No	Yes	Not Applicable
a. Patient-specific parameters for notifying physician of changes in vital signs or other clinical findings	☐ 0	☐ 1	☐ NA Physician has chosen not to establish patient-specific parameters for this patient; agency will use standardized clinical guidelines accessible for all care providers to reference
b. Diabetic foot care including monitoring for the presence of skin lesions on the lower extremities and patient/caregiver education on proper foot care	☐ 0	☐ 1	☐ NA Patient is not diabetic or is bilateral amputee
c. Falls prevention interventions	☐ 0	☐ 1	☐ NA Patient is not assessed to be at risk for falls
d. Depression intervention(s) such as medication, referral for other treatment, or a monitoring plan for current treatment	☐ 0	☐ 1	☐ NA Patient has no diagnosis or symptoms of depression
e. Intervention(s) to monitor and mitigate pain	☐ 0	☐ 1	☐ NA No pain identified
f. Intervention(s) to prevent pressure ulcers	☐ 0	☐ 1	☐ NA Patient is not assessed to be at risk for pressure ulcers

Plan/Intervention	No	Yes	Not Applicable
g. Pressure ulcer treatment based on principles of moist wound healing OR order for treatment based on moist wound healing has been requested from physician	☐ 0	☐ 1	☐ NA Patient has no pressure ulcers with need for moist wound healing

EMERGENT CARE

(M2300) **Emergent Care:** Since the last time OASIS data were collected, has the patient utilized a hospital emergency department (includes holding/observation)?

☐ 0 - No *[Go to M2400]*
☐ 1 - Yes, used hospital emergency department WITHOUT hospital admission
☐ 2 - Yes, used hospital emergency department WITH hospital admission
☐ UK - Unknown *[Go to M2400]*

(M2310) **Reason for Emergent Care**: For what reason(s) did the patient receive emergent care (with or without hospitalization)? **(Mark all that apply.)**

☐ 1 - Improper medication administration, medication side effects, toxicity, anaphylaxis
☐ 2 - Injury caused by fall
☐ 3 - Respiratory infection (e.g., pneumonia, bronchitis)
☐ 4 - Other respiratory problem
☐ 5 - Heart failure (e.g., fluid overload)
☐ 6 - Cardiac dysrhythmia (irregular heartbeat)

☐ 7 - Myocardial infarction or chest pain
☐ 8 - Other heart disease
☐ 9 - Stroke (CVA) or TIA
☐ 10 - Hypo/hyperglycemia, diabetes out of control
☐ 11 - GI bleeding, obstruction, constipation, impaction
☐ 12 - Dehydration, malnutrition
☐ 13 - Urinary tract infection
☐ 14 - IV catheter-related infection or complication
☐ 15 - Wound infection or deterioration
☐ 16 - Uncontrolled pain
☐ 17 - Acute mental/behavioral health problem
☐ 18 - Deep vein thrombosis, pulmonary embolus
☐ 19 - Other than above reasons
☐ UK - Reason unknown

DATA ITEMS COLLECTED AT INPATIENT FACILITY ADMISSION OR AGENCY DISCHARGE ONLY

(M2400) **Intervention Synopsis:** (Check only **one** box in each row.) Since the previous OASIS assessment, were the following interventions BOTH included in the physician-ordered plan of care AND implemented?

Plan/Intervention	No	Yes	Not Applicable
a. Diabetic foot care including monitoring for the presence of skin lesions on the lower extremities and patient/caregiver education on proper foot care	☐ 0	☐ 1	☐ NA Patient is not diabetic or is bilateral amputee

Plan/Intervention	No	Yes	Not Applicable	
b. Falls prevention interventions	☐ 0	☐ 1	☐ NA	Formal multi factor Fall Risk Assessment indicates the patient was not at risk for falls since the last OASIS assessment
c. Depression intervention(s) such as medication, referral for other treatment, or a monitoring plan for current treatment	☐ 0	☐ 1	☐ NA	Formal assessment indicates patient did not meet criteria for depression AND patient did not have diagnosis of depression since the last OASIS assessment
d. Intervention(s) to monitor and mitigate pain	☐ 0	☐ 1	☐ NA	Formal assessment did not indicate pain since the last OASIS assessment
e. Intervention(s) to prevent pressure ulcers	☐ 0	☐ 1	☐ NA	Formal assessment indicates the patient was not at risk of pressure ulcers since the last OASIS assessment
f. Pressure ulcer treatment based on principles of moist wound healing	☐ 0	☐ 1	☐ NA	Dressings that support the principles of moist wound healing not indicated for this patient's pressure ulcers OR patient has no pressure ulcers with need for moist wound healing

(M2410) To which **Inpatient Facility** has the patient been admitted?

☐ 1 - Hospital [*Go to M2430*]
☐ 2 - Rehabilitation facility [*Go to M0903*]
☐ 3 - Nursing home [*Go to M2440*]
☐ 4 - Hospice [*Go to M0903*]
☐ NA - No inpatient facility admission [**Omit "NA" option on TRN.**]

(M2420) **Discharge Disposition:** Where is the patient after discharge from your agency? **(Choose only one answer.)**

☐ 1 - Patient remained in the community (without formal assistive services)
☐ 2 - Patient remained in the community (with formal assistive services)
☐ 3 - Patient transferred to a non institutional hospice
☐ 4 - Unknown because patient moved to a geographic location not served by this agency
☐ UK - Other unknown [*Go to M0903*]

(M2430) **Reason for Hospitalization:** For what reason(s) did the patient require hospitalization? **(Mark all that apply.)**

☐ 1 - Improper medication administration, medication side effects, toxicity, anaphylaxis
☐ 2 - Injury caused by fall
☐ 3 - Respiratory infection (e.g., pneumonia, bronchitis)
☐ 4 - Other respiratory problem
☐ 5 - Heart failure (e.g., fluid overload)
☐ 6 - Cardiac dysrhythmia (irregular heartbeat)
☐ 7 - Myocardial infarction or chest pain
☐ 8 - Other heart disease
☐ 9 - Stroke (CVA) or TIA
☐ 10 - Hypo/hyperglycemia, diabetes out of control

☐ 11 - GI bleeding, obstruction, constipation, impaction
☐ 12 - Dehydration, malnutrition
☐ 13 - Urinary tract infection
☐ 14 - IV catheter-related infection or complication
☐ 15 - Wound infection or deterioration
☐ 16 - Uncontrolled pain
☐ 17 - Acute mental/behavioral health problem
☐ 18 - Deep vein thrombosis, pulmonary embolus
☐ 19 - Scheduled treatment or procedure
☐ 20 - Other than above reasons
☐ UK - Reason unknown *[Go to M0903]*

(M2440) For what **Reason(s)** was the patient **Admitted** to a **Nursing Home?** **(Mark all that apply.)**

☐ 1 - Therapy services
☐ 2 - Respite care
☐ 3 - Hospice care
☐ 4 - Permanent placement
☐ 5 - Unsafe for care at home
☐ 6 - Other
☐ UK - Unknown *[Go to M0903]*

(M0903) **Date of Last (Most Recent) Home Visit:**

__ __ / __ __ / __ __
month/day/year

(M0906) **Discharge/Transfer/Death Date:** Enter the date of the discharge, transfer, or death (at home) of the patient.

__ __ / __ __ / __ __
month/day/year

8

Skilled Nurse Competency Requirements for Home Health Services

Brenda L. Bonham Howe

Registered nurses (RNs) who are self-starting, self-monitoring, and love working independently may find the role of home health nurse very attractive. Most home health organizations prefer applicants with recent medical and surgical experience, skilled at physical assessment, excellent in written and verbal communication skills, and adept at problem solving. Due to the diversity of health problems seen in home health clients, it is important that the nurses recognize knowledge gaps in order to seek additional information or training. Many home health agencies may utilize a competency checklist for self-assessment (see the Appendix to Chapter 7).

Virginia Henderson (1955), often called the "First Lady of Nursing," was a nurse theorist whose definition of nursing espouses the role of home health nursing. She believed that the nurse fills a unique function in the assistance of an individual, sick or well, in the performance of activities that contribute to health, or recovery, or a peaceful death. Henderson identified the elements of basic nursing care as components integrated in helping an individual, where needed, with the following areas:

- Religious and spiritual activities
- Communication associated with needs and feelings
- Performance of appropriate work activities
- Play and recreation
- Learning and human development activities
- Respiration
- Eating and drinking
- Elimination
- Postures and ambulation
- Sleep and rest requirements
- Clothing needs
- Temperature regulation
- Hygiene
- Avoiding danger to self and others (Stizman & Eichelberger, 2011, p. 33)

Components identified in Henderson's list are present in the Medicare Outcome and Assessment Information Set (OASIS) that must be used for all Medicare and Medicaid clients when hospitalized or admitted to a home health service for continuation of skilled care (see the Appendix to Chapter 7). Clients are dependent on accurate assessment and documentation of their health care needs. If documentation does not support the services being given, then Medicare or Medicaid may deny coverage of all or part of the home care support.

EXPECT THE UNEXPECTED

The home health nurse must have the education, experience, and skills to assess clients many miles from a health care facility and possibly without telephone or cell phone access. Situations like this may occur when nurses work in rural areas (Corbet & William, 2014) and must travel great distances between mountains or into canyons. The nurse must be able to assess and make recommendations within nursing's scope of practice, knowing that communication with the primary care provider (PCP) may not occur for an hour or more. It may not be possible to relay the PCP's response before the next day. If the situation dictates, the nurse must advise the client that he or she needs a physician's assessment, and then help to coordinate transportation to the nearest health care facility without conferring with the PCP.

Problem-solving skills are necessary to improvise when there is no access to supplies: A client may need an enema and there is no enema bag or single-unit enema available. The nurse may have a 60 mL irrigation syringe and a single straight catheter kit in her supplies. The catheter may be attached to the end of the syringe for gentle insertion for a tap water enema. Due to the cost of medical supplies, most nurses try to carry a limited quantity of items in their cars, but it is not possible to carry one of everything.

The role of a home health nurse goes beyond that of the "generalist" nurse. Specialty skills include advanced wound care, enterostomal therapy, intravenous infusions, and end-of-life (EOL) care. Home health services go where people live, and may include individuals of every socioeconomic level, every gender preference, every cultural group, and various institutional and correctional facilities. The individual nurse who goes to work in a home health setting must integrate knowledge, abilities, skills, and attitudes to demonstrate competent work performance (Mildon, Betker, & Underwood, 2010).

Home health RN job titles include, but are not limited to, case manager (CM); admissions; on-call; infection control; quality assurance; intake; tele-health coordinator; tele-health staff; clinical educator (CE); foot care nurse; and certified wound, ostomy, and continence nurse (CWOCN).

RN EXPECTATIONS FOR ALL NURSE ROLES

The following list represents characteristic qualifications for many home health nurse roles. Therefore, the list is not repeated with each of the individual job description sections unless specialized training is required. Information is provided by Ken Koenig, Human Resources director at Partners in Care Home Health & Hospice, Bend, OR (2013).

Position Qualifications

- Positive communication and assessment skills
- The ability to use those skills with the client/family, and community providers, including physicians, nurses, social workers, and other professionals
- Graduate of an accredited school of nursing
- One to 2 years of recent medical/surgical care experience in an institutional setting
- One year of home health/hospice care experience preferred
- Program management skills and/or experience preferred
- Current licensure in the state of employment
- Must possess and maintain a current cardiopulmonary resuscitation (CPR) certification
- Must possess and maintain a valid state drivers' license and/or reliable transportation
- Must possess current auto insurance coverage
- Efficient assessment, verbal, problem solving, and written communication skills (see Appendix to Chapter 7).

Intake RN

Job Description

The intake RN is responsible for supporting all aspects of the client intake processes including establishment and maintenance of positive relationships with customers and referral sources.

Essential Job Functions

The intake nurse takes referrals from physicians' offices and requests all necessary information from referral sources. Information is input into the electronic medical records, including verbal orders as needed. Medicare insurance coverage is verified for all referrals. The certification date is verified and copies of the referral sheets are delivered to appropriate persons including medical records, insurance authorization, and scheduling. The intake nurse notifies the nurse when signed physician orders arrive, sends comfort care orders to the physician, and obtains the physician's signature.

Skills Required

- Excellent communication skills
- Computer skill
- Business machine knowledge

Home Health Nurse

Job Description

The home health nurse plans, coordinates, implements, evaluates home health and hospice services, and is experienced in nursing, with an emphasis on community health education. The professional nurse builds from the resources of the organization and community to provide services to meet the needs of individuals and families within their homes. The RN is responsible for cost-efficient and effective client care with quality outcomes.

Essential Job Functions

The home health nurse completes an initial, comprehensive (if home health includes OASIS), and accurate assessment of the client and his or her family to determine home health needs. The nurse provides a complete physical assessment and history of previous illness and uses the health assessment data to determine the appropriate diagnosis and need for other disciplines and resources. An individualized care plan is developed, which establishes goals based on nursing diagnosis and incorporates therapeutic, preventive, and rehabilitative nursing actions. The client and his or her family are included in the planning process.

Ongoing assessments are conducted and the nurse makes necessary revisions to the care plan as the client's status and needs change. Appropriate preventive and rehabilitative nursing procedures and treatments and/or end-of-life comfort measures are initiated. Medications and treatments are administered as prescribed by the physician. Arrangements for equipment and other necessary items and services are available or ordered. A home health aide (HHA) care plan is created as needed and the nurse performs HHA supervisory visits no later than every 14 days. The nurse assesses the need for utilization of a remote patient monitoring device as appropriate to improve clinical efficiency. As a steward of the agency finances, the nurse always considers cost-effective use of supplies/equipment.

The home health nurse provides health care instructions and education to the client and/or family as appropriate as per the assessment plan and the client's caregivers' ability to learn. Teaching styles are adapted to meet client's and family's needs.

The home health nurse identifies discharge-planning needs as part of the initial care plan development, implements them prior to discharge of the client, and adheres to the organization's mission and values.

Communication

- Updates the primary physician when necessary and at least every 60 days

- Communicates with the physician regarding the client's needs and reports any changes in the client's condition; obtains/receives the physician's orders as required
- Communicates with all members of the health care team to promote coordinated, efficient care

Documentation

- Ongoing clinical notes are complete, accurate, documented, and submitted within 24 hours of client visit
- Initial assessments are complete, accurate, and submitted within 48 to 72 hours of admission
- The HHA plan of care is complete, accurate, and updated after every certification or as the client's needs change
- Submits a weekly time sheet that is accurate
- Documents coordination of care with all involved in the client's care

RN–Admissions

Job Description

The admission RN is responsible for admitting clients in accordance with organization policies and procedures. This RN evaluates the client to determine eligibility for home health or hospice.

Essential Job Functions

If a client does not meet criteria for either program, the admission RN offers a transitions program if available and sends the physician a thank-you card for the referral. If the client meets the criteria for home health admission, the nurse reviews the admission packet with the client and/or caregiver and discusses the appropriate program services with the client so that the client and/or caregiver understands and obtains required consents. Then all required documents go to the office for filing in the client's hard-copy chart.

A comprehensive assessment is performed on clients and the initial plan of care. Interventions are planned for pain control and other symptoms as needed. The nurse determines the client's needs for other disciplines and coordinates as needed. Comfort care orders are obtained as appropriate in addition to other medications, supplies, and durable medical equipment (DME). The nurse works collaboratively with the pharmacy, client care coordinator, and physicians to ensure that the client's immediate needs are met.

Instruction is provided by the nurse so that the client and/or caregivers are able to assume care safely until the next nursing visit. Documentation is completed within mandatory time frames so that client information is available to all staff. The nurse reports to the client care coordinator or program director for communication with the interdepartmental team (IDT).

RN–On Call

Job Description

In order to meet the needs of the clients, the on-call RN provides skilled nursing care to the organization clients outside of business hours.

Essential Job Functions

The on-call nurse responds to all calls within 15 minutes of a call from the answering service. The nurse is also responsible for receiving and giving report on clients and/or obtaining client information via e-mail and telephone calls. Visits are made to the clients within 1 hour depending on the location of the client and the acuity level of the visit needed. If the on-call volume is high, the on-call

RN prioritizes visits. The on-call nurse follows the guidelines for making visits as listed in the on-call/weekend services policy.

Physician orders are obtained as needed to provide services/treatments outside the current plan of care. If revisions are made to the plan of care, the on-call RN will inform the nurse CM by phone or e-mail. The nurse completes all necessary documentation as per RN guidelines and time frames. Attendance at IDT and case conferences is appropriate or a detailed report to the client care coordinator or program director is necessary.

The weekend 24-hour position is the primary on-call position and this nurse coordinates all client visit/call activity with the secondary 12-hour on-call position. The weeknight on-call position has the sole responsibility of coordinating all client visits/call activities.

RN Case Manager

Job Description

The RN CM plans, coordinates, implements, evaluates home health and hospice services, and is experienced in nursing, with an emphasis on community health education. The CM builds from the resources of the organization and community to provide services to meet the needs of individuals and families within their homes. The CM is responsible for cost-efficient and effective client care with quality outcomes.

Essential Job Functions

An initial comprehensive and accurate assessment (OASIS) of client and family is done to determine health care needs. A complete physical assessment and history of previous illness(es) using the health assessment data will determine appropriate diagnosis and need for other disciplines and resources. An individualized care plan is developed, which establishes goals based on nursing diagnosis and incorporates therapeutic, preventive, and rehabilitative nursing actions. If an HHA is appropriate the nurse develops a care plan for the HHA and provides supervisory visits no later than every 14 days. The client and the family are included in the planning process. Arrangements are made for equipment, medications, and other necessary items and services as per availability. Ongoing assessments are completed, and the care plan is updated as the client's status changes.

The nurse performs procedures and treatments and/or end-of-life comfort measures according to the plan of care. Medications and treatments are administered as prescribed by the physician. Health care instructions and education are provided to the client and/or family as appropriate according to the assessment plan and client's and/or caregiver's ability to learn. The teaching styles are adapted to meet the client's and his or her family's needs.

Tele-Health Coordinator

Job Description

The tele-health coordinator implements and builds community awareness for the remote patient monitor program, and is responsible for program efficiency/performance and effectiveness. Statistical information on program is updated and copies given to the program director as needed. Staff awareness is refreshed about the efficient use of T-Monitor systems. The tele-health coordinator supervises installation and maintenance of T-Monitors and central station staff. Proactive marketing techniques are utilized to promote the program to target groups of physicians and customers.

RN–Remote Patient Monitoring

Job Description

The central station clinician utilizes remote patient monitoring to review clients' vital sign trends and provides appropriate follow-up with care managers and/or physicians and completes accurate and timely documentation.

Essential Job Functions

Data alerts are reviewed for abnormal parameters and the RN communicates with the client regarding the status. Abnormal parameters are evaluated and the nurse uses clinical judgment to determine if the client's physician should be contacted. New orders are entered into the clinical documentation record and the client is notified and educated regarding the change. The client's nurse CM is also notified by phone or through secured e-mail. If the nurse determines that the client's physician does not need to be contacted, the client is given appropriate instructions or reassurances. Coordination with the nurse CM ensures continuity of care. The nurse sends T-Monitor trend reports to the physicians and nurse CM as appropriate or requested.

RN–Triage

Job Description

The triage RN works in coordination with on-call RNs to provide on-call nursing services to organization clients outside of business hours.

Essential Job Functions

The triage RN will respond to all client calls within 5 to 10 minutes of the call from the answering service. It is important to have access to the client's chart to verify medications and plan of care. Interventions are provided over the phone whenever possible with a status-check call within 30 minutes. If there is a need for an on-call nursing visit, the on-call nurse is notified. If a visit is not needed, the triage nurse will obtain physician orders when needed and will update the medication list. Necessary prescriptions are coordinated with the pharmacy. New DME delivery is arranged through a medical equipment supplier. Any necessary changes are made to the plan of care and the nurse CM is notified by phone or secure e-mail.

New referrals that require an admission on the weekend are prioritized and on-call RNs are notified. The weekend triage nurse communicates with the intake nurse with regard to referrals for Monday admissions.

Wound, Ostomy, Continence Nurse

Job Description

The wound, ostomy, continence nurse (WOCN) provides care in the home setting and community to clients with ostomies, draining wounds, fistulas, pressure ulcers, acute or chronic wounds, and continence disorders. The WOCN acts as a consultant and educator to the clinical staff.

Essential Job Functions

The WOCN provides a valuable service to clients and the home health organization. Consultation and assistance are provided to staff in the development and implementation of protocols used in the identification and management of clients with potential or actual alteration in skin integrity. The WOCN collaborates with nurse CMs on development of individualized care plans that establish appropriate, measurable goals for clients with complex, nonhealing wounds, incontinence, and ostomy problems. Collaboration with nurse CMs is key in the evaluation of the clients' responses to treatment. Care plans are updated when adjustments or modifications are indicated.

The WOCN evaluates, selects, and recommends supplies and equipment for clients with ostomies, wounds, fistulas, pressure ulcers, and continence care to ensure efficacy and cost effectiveness of products used for skin and wound care. Consultation with sales representatives provides the WOCN with information on the development and maintenance of a formulary of stock items and purchasing contracts to ensure the most cost-effective and efficient use of wound and ostomy supplies.

Health care instruction and education provision is a vital aspect of the WOCN professional role. It is important for the client and his or her family to understand the goals set in the client's healing or recovery. It is important that the WOCN is knowledgeable in adapting the teaching style to meet the client's needs.

The WOCN provides appropriate debridement of devitalized tissues (conservative sharp debridement; silver nitrate cauterization of nonproliferative wound edges, removal of hypertrophic granulation tissues, and control of minor bleeding). It is important to note that the WOCN's scope may vary from state to state. The WOCN communicates with all members of the health care team, including the physician, to coordinate the care plan related to wound, ostomy, and continence needs. All appropriate documentation is completed in the established time frame of 48 to 72 hours.

Position Qualifications

- Graduate from an accredited WOCN education program
- Two years RN experience
- BS or BSN preferred
- Possessing and maintaining a current CPR card
- Current RN state license
- WOCN certification by WOCN board

Clinical Educator

Job Description

The CE is responsible for ensuring the overall clinical competency of the nursing staff. This includes clinical orientation of new nursing staff and mentoring of existing nursing staff.

Essential Job Functions

The CE utilizes the initial competency assessment skills checklist, assesses the competency of all new nursing staff, and arranges mentoring as needed to ensure proficiency. Home visits are coordinated with nursing staff prior to the 90-day or annual review to ensure clinical competency.

The CE plans and coordinates in-services/education for clinical staff and also assists in provision of educational tools for clients. The CE sends out an annual survey for all staff skills self-assessment and requests for educational in-services. The CE develops the annual education plan for professional and support staff based on needs assessment. An annual safety and skills lab review is organized with review topics included that are appropriate for all employees.

Skills Required

- Demonstrates an ability to work with health care clinicians
- Self-directed and able to work with minimal supervision
- Background in teaching or education is desirable
- Able to adapt teaching methods to learners
- Demonstrates excellent observation, verbal, and written communication skills
- Possesses excellent clinical nursing skills

Foot Care RN

Job Description

The foot care registered nurse (FCRN) is responsible for organization and supervision of foot care clinics and for foot care provided to clients who are unable to leave their homes.

Essential Job Functions

The FCRN is responsible for efficiency and cost effectiveness of foot clinics and supervises foot clinic staff. As the supervisor for this service, the FCRN develops and updates policies and procedures, orders and maintains foot care supplies, and oversees collection and receipt of payment.

The FCRN supervises foot care staff and ensures that proper assessment and documentation are provided to clients. Foot care education information for clients is kept current and available. Referrals are made to podiatrists as appropriate, as the foot care staff works within its scope of practice and education.

Skills Required

- Education and experience to work in the FCRN scope as defined by the State Board of Nursing
- Ability to work independently
- Ability to organize and coordinate foot care clinics
- Ability to supervise others
- Ability to work with a variety of health care providers

Home Health Nursing Supervisor

Job Description

The home health nursing supervisor is responsible for day-to-day supervision of home health clinical staff and processes to ensure quality client care and outcomes.

Essential Job Function

The supervisor assists the scheduler as needed to assign home health clients to the appropriate clinician based on geographic location;

client's needs; and the clinician's expertise, abilities, and caseload. The supervisor ensures the clinical competency of the staff by mentoring, reviewing documentation, attending case conferences, and home visits. Professionalism and excellent customer service are encouraged in addition to demonstrating concern with promotion of staff satisfaction. The supervisor provides useful developmental feedback and may need to implement a corrective action plan with staff to address performance and other issues. Incident reporting and follow-up are done by the supervisor, who uses the opportunity for staff education for those involved in the situation. The supervisor assists in the interviewing and hiring process of new professional staff and takes part in the orientation process by collaboration with the CE. Supervision and evaluation of new staff are provided within 90 days of hire. The supervisor also reviews staff productivity and documentation timelines.

The supervisor may also participate in the organization's committees—budget committee, safety committee, community outreach—and other duties delegated by the clinical operations director.

Home Health Program Coordinator

Job Description

The home health program coordinator (HHPC) is a professional nurse responsible for coding and analyzing data integrity and consistency of OASIS documentation and assessment processes. The HHPC is responsible for ensuring positive clinical and financial outcomes for the home health program. He or she ensures regulatory compliance and program efficacy.

Essential Job Functions

The HHPC prospectively reviews all OASIS assessments to ensure appropriateness, completeness, and compliance with federal and state regulations and organization policy. The HHPC utilizes OASIS variation or alert reports when reviewing OASIS data and ensures appropriate International Classification of Diseases-10 (ICD-10) coding and sequencing as it relates to the client's medical condition. The HHPC serves as a regulatory specialist for home health and assists staff to adhere to all regulatory criteria with the inclusion of admission to service and ongoing coverage.

The HHPC assists in the formulation, revision, implementation, and evaluation of home health policies, procedures, and strategic goals. The HHPC reviews visit utilization for appropriateness of care guidelines and client condition and reports potential financial losses and/or underutilization to the nursing supervisor and clinical operations director. The HHPC notifies the home health nursing supervisor and clinical operations director of problematic trends as a result of the OASIS review. Participation in committees includes quality improvement and corporate compliance review. It is important for the HHPC to maintain professional and technical knowledge by the attendance of educational workshops and the review of professional publications as related to Medicare OASIS-C.

Infection Control Nurse

Job Description

The infection control nurse (ICN) is responsible for implementing and maintaining an effective infection control program that protects clients, families, and organization personnel by preventing and controlling infections and communicable diseases.

Essential Job Functions

The ICN oversees the regular review and update of organization infection control policies and conducts infection control classes on an annual basis for organization staff. Immunization status is tracked for new and existing staff. It is expected that the ICN participates in the safety committee and takes part in new employee safety orientation. If flu shot clinics are held by the organization, the ICN plans and coordinates the event.

Skills Required

- Strong organizational skills
- Ability to work independently with minimal supervision
- Strong oral and written communications skills

Quality Coordinator

Job Description

The quality coordinator (QC; CMS, 2010) is responsible for tracking and maintaining all of the home health and hospice quality activities of the organization. The QC acts as the infection coordinator and is responsible for implementing and maintaining an effective infection control program that protects clients, families, and agency personnel by preventing and controlling infections and communicable diseases.

Essential Job Functions

The QC provides direction and coordination of quality improvement activities utilizing continuous quality improvement principles and methodologies. The QC coordinates activities related to clinical record review of data collection and compiling trends and reports of quality data in the following areas: client care and outcomes, client and staff infection control, safety, and other areas in collaboration with the quality compliance director.

All infection reports are reviewed for completeness, risk, standard of care determination, and appropriate follow-up, and logged for trending. The QC collaborates with clinical supervisors to provide a process to promote and ensure employee orientation, competency, and in-service and education programs for both the quality and infection control programs. As a clinical resource to staff regarding quality issues and infection control, the QC assists in the identification of skills for annual competence and provides in-service training support.

SUMMARY

- Home health nurses provide a holistic care service because they work with the client in the usual home environment. Family and client are included in decision making related to the plan of care.
- RNs work in a variety of roles with home health care services.
- Flexibility is key for the home health nurse, as working away from a facility makes the work environment much more unpredictable.
- Critical thinking skills are important for problem solving independently.
- Being a home health nurse is a complex and demanding role. There is a high turnover and anyone who is considering home health work needs to research the topic. It is not an easy job and may lead to very long workdays. Unlike a facility, where work hours may be posted 8 a.m. to 5 p.m., a home health nurse is given an assignment for the day. The nurse works until those clients are seen, regardless of phone calls, flat tires, or miles driven between visits. "Always expect the unexpected" is an excellent motto for a home health nurse. What one may think is a simple visit may include unexpected complications and a delay in the day's schedule. Work for the day is not complete until all documentation is complete. First- and last-visit OASIS assessment documentation may take 1.5 to 2 hours. All necessary phone, fax, or e-mail contacts must be made before the lights go out.
- Home health nursing has many positive rewards in spite of the challenges.

RESOURCES

Home Health Nurses Association

http://www.hhna.org

Search Terms
- Overview
- Mission
- Resources

National Association of Home Care

http://www.nahc.org

Search Terms
- Caring
- Advocacy and policy
- Resources and services

REFERENCES

Centers for Medicare and Medicaid Services (CMS). *Home health quality initiative: OASIS-C 2012*. Retrieved May 10, 2014, from http://www.cms.gov/Medicare/Quality-Initiatives-Client-AssessmentInstruments/HomeHealthQualityInits/Downloads/HHQIOASISCAllTimePoint.pdf

Corbet, S., & William, F. (2014). Striking balance: Interactions between nurses and their older rural clients. *British Journal of Community Nursing*, 19(4), 162–167.

Mildon, B., Betker, C., & Underwood, J. (2010). Standards of practice in community health nursing: A literature review undertaken to inform revisions to the Canadian Community Health Nursing Standards of Practice. Community Health Nurses of Canada. Retrieved September 2014 from http://www.chnc.ca/documents/ALitReviewUndertakentoInformRevisionstotheCdnCHNStdofPracticeMarch2011.pdf

Stizman, K., & Eichelberger, L. W. (2011). *Understanding the work of nurse theorists: A creative beginning*. Sudbury, MA: Jones & Bartlett Publishers.

9

Hospice and Palliative Care Services

Stephanie Bernahl Barss

END-OF-LIFE CARE

There is no one way to provide end-of-life care. Hospice services are for people who have a serious illness and can be offered in a variety of settings ranging from a person's home to a clinical inpatient unit such as a hospital or nursing home (Friedrich, 1999). In addition, end-of-life care will "look" different depending on which part of the country you live in. In this chapter, we explore hospice and palliative care as well as trends and opportunities within the industry (Moyer, Moyer, Pallet, & Mannes, 2000).

THE START OF HOSPICE

In 1982, the federal government made a provision for the Medicare hospice benefit. This provision became permanent in 1986 entitling every eligible citizen access to hospice care (Department of Health and Human Services, 2013). Hospice services are provided though the Centers for Medicare and Medicaid Services (CMS); however, for individuals not eligible for Medicare, state and private insurances will often pay for a portion of the hospice costs and many hospices will provide services at a reduced rate or free of charge (Gerace, 2013).

WHO IS ELIGIBLE FOR MEDICARE HOSPICE BENEFITS?

In order to be considered "eligible" for hospice one must meet the following conditions (CMS, 2013):

- The client is eligible for Medicare Part A
- A doctor and the hospice medical director certify that the client has a life-limiting illness and death is expected in 6 months or less
- The client signs a statement giving permission to choose hospice care instead of other Medicare-covered benefits (Medicare will still cover health problems not related to the terminal prognosis)
- Client enrolls in a Medicare-approved hospice program (Hospice Medicine Foundation, n.d.)

WHAT IS HOSPICE CARE?

Hospice is holistic care at the end of life. It is offered to people and their families facing a life-limiting terminal illness. It provides medical, emotional, spiritual, and functional support. Care is provided based on the patient's individual needs and wishes (Friedrich, 1999). The goals and interventions are developed directly by the patient and the interdisciplinary team (IDT). Often goals are related to symptom management, psychological or emotional needs, and spiritual processes. Once a patient has elected the hospice benefit the hospice agency is responsible to provide core services and in turn pays for the care related to the terminal diagnosis. Hospice care can be provided in any location—a home, facility, or inpatient care setting. Support is also provided to the patient's loved ones during the course of illness and after the patient's death via bereavement for up to 12 months (National Hospice and Palliative Care Organization [NHPCO], 2013a).

THE IDT

Hospice care services are provided by a team of experts known as the IDT. The core people who provide care include medical professionals (doctors, advanced practice nurses, pharmacists, and nurses), social workers, and spiritual counselors (Figure 9.1). There are a number of other specialist members of the IDT who are available to support patients and families (similar to the home health team noted in the previous chapter) and include certified home health aides, therapists (physical, occupational, nutrition, speech, bereavement, pet, music, acupuncture, massage), and volunteers (Standard of Practice for Hospice Programs, 2010).

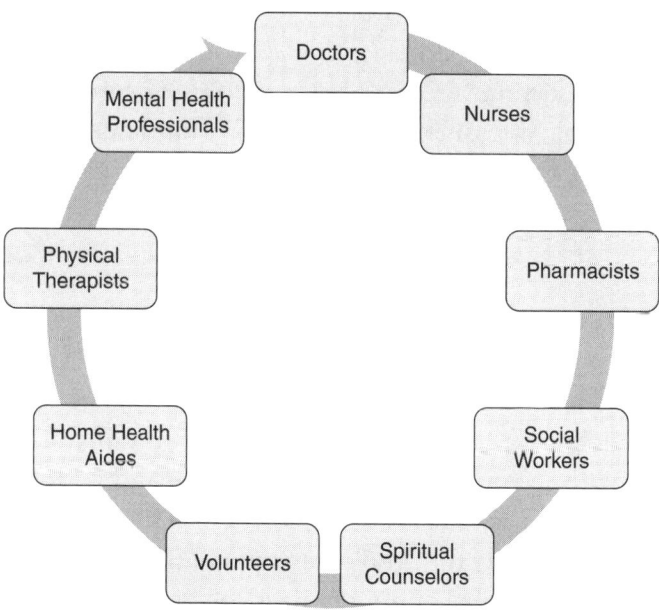

FIGURE 9.1   Interdisciplinary team (IDT).

HOW IS HOSPICE SERVICE INITIATED?

First, hospice is ordered by a physician who determines that a patient has a terminal illness with a life expectancy of 6 months or less if the disease runs its normal course. Once this initial referral is made, the hospice medical director will certify the patient indeed meets the eligibility requirements mandated by Medicare. Finally, a specially trained hospice nurse will be dispatched for an assessment and the formal signing of terms and conditions of admission.

The hospice nurse completes a thorough assessment. The Outcome and Assessment Instrument Set (OASIS) template used for home health is also used for hospice patients (see the Appendix to Chapter 7). However, there are some variations as to documentation requirements. There are also two end-of-life assessment tools. Some of the common scales used in hospice and palliative care may be found at Hospice Medicine Foundation Organization (see the References section):

- Palliative Performance Scale
- Karnofsky Performance Status
- Eastern Cooperative Oncology Group (ECOG) for cancer patients
- Functional Assessment Staging (FAST) for dementia patients
- New York Heart Association (NYHA) class for congestive heart failure patients

WHAT TO EXPECT ON HOSPICE?

At the center of the hospice philosophy is the belief that each of us has the right to die free of pain and with dignity. Care is also provided with the goal of comfort versus cure and with an emphasis on quality of life. The focus is patient and family centered and takes care to support the whole person, not just the disease. Once enrolled on hospice, an individualized plan of care is developed, which helps guide the team to best support the patient and family during the days, weeks, and months ahead. This plan is revisited and adapted frequently as needed.

Typically, the day-to-day care is provided by a family member. Patients who are exceptionally debilitated may also have support provided by paid caregivers either in their own home or in a home-like setting such as a foster home, assisted living, or nursing home (these services are not part of the hospice benefit). The hospice team is not in place of caregivers; rather, they add another layer of support providing expertise to help better manage the patient's symptoms and concerns. Individual hospice team members make visits depending on individual patient needs and wants. A hospice registered nurse (RN) is on call 24 hours a day, 7 days a week.

The care of hospice patients may include the following (Nabili, n.d):

- Managing evolving medical issues (infections, medication management, pressure ulcers, hydration, nutrition, physical stages of dying)
- Treating physical symptoms (pain, shortness of breath, anxiety, nausea, vomiting, constipation, confusion, etc.)
- Counseling about the anxiety, uncertainty, grief, and fear associated with end of life and dying
- Providing support to patients, their families, and caregivers with the overwhelming physical and psychological stresses of a terminal illness
- Guiding patients and families through the difficult interpersonal and psychosocial issues and helping them with finding closure
- Paying attention to personal, religious, spiritual, and cultural values
- Assisting patients and families reaching financial closures (living will, trust, advance directive, funeral arrangements)
- Providing bereavement counseling to the mourning loved ones after the death of the patient

FUNDING AND FINANCIAL ISSUES

Today the number of hospice organizations exceeds 5,500 nationwide and operate as part of a hospital system, home health agency, nursing home, or are freestanding and independent (NHPCO, 2013a). Furthermore, according to NHPCO, each hospice organization falls into one of three tax categories:

1. Not-for-profit (charitable organizations): 32%
2. For-profit (the majority of hospices fall into this category): 63%
3. Government owned: 5%

As you read this, the hospice as we know it is at risk. The industry is facing increased government regulation and significant cuts in hospice reimbursement. Unfortunately, this is happening as health care costs are rising and the population is aging (many of whom will soon qualify for hospice services). It is broadly understood and research shows that hospice use saves money and reduces Medicare program expenditure (National Consensus Project for Quality Palliative Care, 2013). However, there is concern among hospice professionals that the government revisions threaten the vitality of hospice as we know it.

PALLIATIVE CARE

Palliative care is expanded from the hospice model. Palliative care aims to help support individuals who have a life-limiting illness but whose life expectancy is more than 6 months and may still be pursuing treatment and cure (NHPCO, 2013b). Currently, hospice services are provided to people who are eligible based on the guidelines set by Medicare, but palliative care services are not directly reimbursed by Medicare Part A nor are they controlled and regulated as rigorously as hospice. Palliative care can be offered to individuals at any age or stage of illness. NHPCO's

Standards of Practice for Hospice Programs (2010) describe palliative care as:

> Treatment that enhances comfort and improves the quality of an individual's life during the last phase of life. No specific therapy is excluded from consideration. The individual choices and decisions regarding care are paramount and must be followed.

Palliative care teams are being organized in inpatient and outpatient settings around the country. The specific services provided by palliative care professionals are similar to hospice services, but are more generalized. Examples of common palliative care referrals according to the NHPCO link to the page for Caring Connections (www.caringinfo.org) are:

- Patient/family/provider needs help with complex treatment decision making
- Support for suffering and/or other symptoms of distress
- Prolonged hospital stays without evidence of improvement
- An intensive care unit (ICU) patient with documented poor prognosis
- Withdrawal of life support in the ICU
- Care of the dying patient and support of the family
- Assistance to determine hospice eligibility and referral

Palliative care grew from the needs of patients who have complex symptoms related to their illness, yet their life expectancy is more than 6 months but typically less than 5 years. Palliative care can help patients and families work on advance care planning, living wills, goals of care, and symptom management.

CONCLUSION

Hospice and palliative care remain underutilized. The reasons are varied. In our culture it is not easy to talk of dying and death. In the United States, there persists an avoidance of speaking about advanced illness, dying, and grief. The subject of death remains taboo. Physicians have long been trained to save life at all cost and see death as the enemy (Moyer et al., 2000). Forty percent of people still die in hospital ICUs (Smith, Mir, & Lahaj, 2011). Furthermore, cultural differences among people impact exposure and admission to hospice and palliative care programs. The access is limited by the inappropriate delivery in clinical settings and acceptance by individuals within specific ethnic groups. Some people believe that merely talking about dying invites death or others consider discussion about dying a sign of disrespect and insensitivity (Brandt, Abuadude, Canuteson, Radulovic, & Merrman, 2013). Hospice and palliative care provide a culturally sensitive network of trained professionals who specialize in supporting patients, families, communities, and other health professionals who grapple with the complex issues presented as we near end of life. Hospice and palliative care specialists can help facilitate conversations. And talk we must. Talk will not hasten death, but we must talk in order to provide the opportunity for better deaths for many more Americans (Wright, 2008). Offering hospice and palliative care consults sooner to patients who have complex diseases will give them more time to repair, mend, and heal, moving toward death with the grace, dignity, and peace that each of us deserves.

SUMMARY

- There are many options for end-of-life care. Standardized hospice care is one choice that is available in the United States.
- The federal government made a provision for the Medicare hospice benefit in 1982.
- Medicare sets the guidelines for hospice eligibility.
- The IDT of the hospice service reviews goals and interventions for each client. Team members include the client and family,

doctors, advanced practice nurses, pharmacists, nurses, social workers, spiritual counselors, and additional members as needed (hospice aide, physical therapist, occupational therapist, nutritional counsel, speech therapist, pet therapist, and volunteers).
- Hospice support includes (but is not limited to) respect of the individual and personal choices, relief from symptoms and pain, management for evolving medical issues that the individual is at risk of, support and guidance for family and close friends, assistance with financial closures, and bereavement counseling.
- Hospice organizations may include those not for profit, for profit, and government owned.
- Palliative care allows the individual and physician to explore and utilize potential life-extending therapy, which is not included in hospice service.

RESOURCES

Byock, I. (1997). *Dying well: The prospect for growth at the end of life.* New York, NY: Putnam/Riverhead Books.

Ross-Kübler, E. (1969). *On death and dying.* New York, NY: Simon and Schuster.

Aging With Dignity

http://www.agingwithdignity.org/forms/5wishes.pdf

Search Terms
- Five Wishes
- What is Five Wishes?
- Who will make decisions for me when I cannot?
- What kind of treatment do I want?
- How comfortable do I want to be?

National Hospice and Palliative Care Organization

www.NHPCO.org

Search Terms
- About NHPCO
- Membership
- Advocacy
- Education
- Regulatory
- Quality
- Resources

REFERENCES

Brandt, K., Abuadude, M., Canuteson, S., Radulovic, J., & Merrman, M. (2013). *Private conversations and public discourse. Caring connections.* Retrieved from http://www.caringinfo.org/files/public/PrivateConversations_and_PublicDiscourse.pdf.

Centers for Medicare and Medicaid Services (CMS). (2013). *Medicare hospice benefits.* Retrieved October 28, 2013, from http://www.medicare.gov/pubs/pdf/02154.pdf

Department of Health and Human Services (DHHS). (2013). Retrieved October 13, 2013, from http://oig.hhs.gov/oei/reports/oei-02-06-00223.pdf

Friedrich, M. J. (1999). Hospice care in the United States: A conversation with Florence S. Wald. *JAMA: Journal of the American Medical Association, 281,* 1683–1685.

Gerace, A. (March 14, 2013). *Hospice care enrollment saves millions in Medicare dollars.* Retrieved from http://homehealthcarenews.com/2013/03/hospice-care-enrollment-saves-millions-in-medicare-dollars

Hospice Medicine Foundation. (n.d.). *Assessment of functional status.* Retrieved May 18, 2014, from http://www.hospicemedicinefoundation.org/educational-material/assessment-of-functional-status

Moyer, B., Moyer J. D., Pallett, G., & Mannes, E. (2000). *On our own terms.* Arlington, VA: PBS.

Nabili, S. (n.d). *Hospice*. Retrieved November 8, 2013, from http://www.medicinenet.com/hospice

National Consensus Project for Quality Palliative Care. (2013). *Clinical practice guidelines for quality palliative care* (3rd ed.). Pittsburg, PA: Editor Constance Dahlin.

National Hospice and Palliative Care Organization (NHPCO). (2014). *Caring connection*. Retrieved October 2, 2013, from http://www.caringinfo.org.

National Hospice and Palliative Care Organization (NHPCO). (n.d.). *History of hospice care*. Retrieved October 2, 2013, from http://www.nhpco.org/history-hospice-care

National Hospice and Palliative Care Organization (NHPCO). (2013a edition). *NHPCO facts and figures: Hospice care in America*. Retrieved May 2014, from www.nhpco.org/sites/default/files/public/Statistics_Research/2013_Facts_Figures.pdf

National Hospice and Palliative Care Organization (NHPCO). (2013b). *Palliative care*. Retrieved April from http://www.nhpco.org/palliative-care

Rierden, A. (1998, April 19). *A calling for care of the terminally ill*. New York Times. Retrieved November 1, 2013, from http://www.nytimes.com/1998/04/19/nyregion/a-calling-for-care-of-the-terminally-ill.html?pagewanted=all&src=pm

Smith, F., Mir, T., & Lahaj, M. (2011). *Palliative care and hospice: A panel discussion*. Retrieved April 2014, from http://jima.imana.org/article/viewFile/9209/43-3_9

Standard of Practice for Hospice Programs (SPHP). (2010). Retrieved from http://www.nhpco.org/sites/default/files/public/quality/Standards/NHPCO_STANDARDS_2010CD.pdf

Wright, A. A., Zhang, B., Ray, A., Mack, J. W., Trice, E., Balboni, T,... Prigerson, H. G. (2008). Associations between end-of-life discussions, patient mental health, medical care near death, and caregiver bereavement adjustment. *JAMA: Journal of American Medical Association, 300*, 1665–1667.

10

Skilled Nurse Competency Requirements for Hospice Services

Brenda L. Bonham Howe

To consider the differences between the roles of the home health nurse and the hospice nurse, it is best to consider how home health and hospice services vary. First, the purpose of home health is usually rehabilitative with goals set to promote healing, mobility, and as much independence as possible for the client. Next, hospice is a service provided to individuals who may have 6 months or less to live. The focus of hospice care is symptom relief and quality of life; therefore the care plan will be based on needs associated with the terminal diagnosis.

    The variable occurs when a client on home health fails to improve and may fit the criteria appropriate for hospice. The client or family members may not be willing to accept hospice support. The client may still require skilled medical management by a nurse. In that case, home health service may continue as long as the client meets the recertification requirements. The home health nurse then has the opportunity to gently educate the client and family about the benefits of hospice (which may mean dispelling myths).

Hospice nurses provide much of the same care and demonstrate the same variety of skills as home health nurses (see Chapter 8 for a home health nurse job description). Many nurses begin their hospice career by obtaining a year or more in a hospital medical unit or intensive care unit (ICU). In those work settings, they learn about serious and critical health symptoms in addition to symptom management. Additional hospice skills are learned on the job and through continuing education with the exception of the "personal touch."

What is the "personal touch" that many nurses are capable of giving to their clients? The personal touch may be described in many ways. It is based in part on the client's perception and expectations of the staff (Asadi-Lari, Tamburini, & Gray, 2004). The nurse's observable level of comfort in providing care to someone who has been given a terminal diagnosis no doubt allays some of the client's concerns. It is important for the nurse to be at ease and to respond professionally as the client or family demonstrates the highs and lows of their grief process. Perhaps it is utilizing a "sixth sense" that enables recognition of some of the patient's needs described in *Gordon's Functional Health Patterns* (Koshar, n.d.). The best personal touch any nurse can give to any client is that of being present in the moment. Taking the time to be present forges a sense of trust in the hospice nurse at a very vulnerable time in the lives of the client and family members.

The hospice nurse collaborates with other team members, including the medical social worker and spiritual support person. Communicating with the other team members to update them after a visit (by phone or secure e-mail) promotes continuity of care. Occasionally, joint visits by the nurse and social worker or nurse and spiritual support person may provide some new insights into the client's or family's needs.

WHAT TO EXPECT WHEN THE END COMES

The hospice nurse must help to prepare the client and family members for what is to come when they are willing and ready to talk about that part of the journey. Although the future cannot be perfectly predicted, there are many questions that may be answered. The hospice nurse may reassure the clients that support staff will always be available to respond by phone or personal visit. How the end may come depends on the terminal diagnosis. Many clients gradually fade into a coma. The hospice nurse than educates the family or caregivers about how to care for someone in a coma.

With some diseases, organ failure may contribute to bleeding out. This can be very distressing to family members especially if they have no knowledge that it may occur. If there is a potential for bleeding out, it is a good idea to coordinate with the family and agency to obtain some red or brown sheets and towels. Use of the darker color simply neutralizes the shock factor that pools of blood may produce.

HOSPICE NURSES ARE ETERNAL STUDENTS OF HUMAN NATURE

Hospice nurses must be detail oriented and proficient in reading human actions, interactions, and reactions. To keep skills sharp, it is important to practice. To improve skills, it is important to learn new information and to be in touch with current trends in health care. One of the best ways a hospice nurse may do this is by participation in a professional organization. Certification and professional affiliation help to validate the competence of the members.

NATIONAL HOSPICE AND PALLIATIVE CARE ORGANIZATION

The National Hospice and Palliative Care Organization (NHPCO, 2014) sets the standards for quality care and service in the United States. The website includes links to webinars and online education opportunities.

In addition to promotion of proactive continuing education, agency membership creates a partnership for excellence of service, excellence of care, and excellence of positive outcomes for families of hospice clients. NHPCO provides resources for quality improvement, performance measures, and staffing guideline considerations.

The NHPCO lists 10 components of quality in hospice care applicable to the role of hospice nurse.

1. Patient- and family-centered care
2. Ethical behavior and computer rights
3. Clinical excellence and safety
4. Inclusion and access
5. Organizational excellence
6. Workforce excellence
7. Standards
8. Compliance with laws and regulations
9. Stewardship and accountability
10. Performance measurement

NATIONAL BOARD FOR CERTIFICATION OF HOSPICE AND PALLIATIVE CARE NURSES

The National Board for Certification of Hospice and Palliative Care Nurses (NBCHPN) is the only organization that offers certificaiton to hospice and palliative care nurses. Each certification is valid for a 4-year period, after which the nurse may renew the credential. Currently, the NBCHPN certifies more than 18,000 health professionals. The mission of the NBCHPN is, "To advance expert care in serious illness through a focus on continuing competence" (NBCHPN, 2014).

SUMMARY

- Skills required for home health or hospice may vary slightly based on projected outcomes.

- Home health focuses on rehabilitation and restoration of health status and hospice focuses on end-of-life and comfort care.
- Nurses are educated to provide compassionate care in all settings.
- Hospice nurses are prepared to work with clients and families through the grief process.
- Hospice nurses provide oversight and teach caregivers about comfort control measures and pain management in addition to guidance through the signs and symptoms of the dying process.
- The NHPCO sets standards for quality care and service in the United States. Membership may be preferred by hospice employers because it indicates that the nurse has passed a national certification test.

RESOURCES

Callanan, M., & Kelley, P. (1997). *Final gifts: Understanding the special awareness, needs, and communications of the dying.* New York, NY: Bantam-Dell.
CHPN study guide. (2014). Trivium Test Prep.

Hospice Foundation of America

http://www.hospicefoundation.org/endoflife

Search Terms
- Myths about dying
- Signs of approaching death
- Advance care planning
- What to expect after death
- Pain and patient comfort

REFERENCES

Asadi-Lari, M., Tamburini, M., & Gray, D. (2004). Patients' needs, satisfaction, and health related quality of life: Towards a comprehensive model. *Health Quality Life Outcomes, 2,* 32. Published online June 29, 2004. Retrieved May 21, 2014, from http://www.ncbi.nlm.nih.gov/pmc/articles/PMC471563

Koshar, J. (n.d.). *Gordon's functional health patterns. Course 340 women's health & illness in the expanding family.* Retrieved May 20, 2014, from http://www.sonoma.edu/ users/k/koshar/n340/n345_NANDA.html

National Board for Certification of Hospice and Palliative Nurses (NBCHPN). (2014). *Welcome homepage.* Retrieved May 21, 2014, from http://www.nbchpn.org

National Hospice and Palliative Care Organization (NHPCO). (2014). *About NHPCO.* Retrieved May 21, 2014, from http://www.nhpco.org

11

Independent Living

Brenda L. Bonham Howe

WHAT IS INDEPENDENT LIVING?

Independent living usually refers to a retirement community where people 55 years and older choose to live for convenience and socialization opportunities. Residents are in general good health and do not require supervision as they go about their daily routines. They are responsible for taking their own medications as well as making their own medical appointments. If minimal assistance is needed, then the resident is responsible for making those arrangements with medical management support from a home health or home care agency (Robinson, Saisan, & White, 2014).

AMENITIES

Retirement communities usually offer a number of amenities that help to attract people to a lifestyle where they are able to enjoy more free time. Benefits associated with retirement communities include a choice of smaller home or condominium style of living, which reduces housekeeping chores. Often utilities, including electricity, water, sewer, and garbage disposal, are included in the cost. Sometimes housekeeping is included with specific responsibilities. Home maintenance or lawn and garden care may be provided by facility employees or contracted services. Additional options may include a parking space, storage, and a pet agreement. Sometimes the retirement community leases space for onsite businesses such as a beauty salon, barber, bank, and restaurant, which adds to the convenience and feeling of a contained community of friends and acquaintances (Howell, 2014).

ACTIVITIES

Recreational opportunities are common and may include putting greens, walking trails, outdoor gardening space with a hothouse, arts and crafts, fitness center, and auditorium for guest entertainers, and planned movie nights. Transportation may also be part of the community amenities. Buses or vans are often available to take scheduled trips to specific malls, churches, libraries, or sightseeing tours. There may also be a resident's relations/concierge service to assist with activity planning.

Lifelong learning is recognized as an important aspect of keeping the brain active and engaged in information that goes beyond the living space. The purpose is to expand and enrich individuals by providing space for study groups; arts and crafts; and outings to fairs, exhibits, and concerts.

Intergenerational opportunities may be planned with youth clubs or school groups. One example observed by the author was a home-schooling group of six students who read short stories they had written, played musical instruments, and sang a group song. The residents then served the students cookies and punch and spent time visiting with them. The students felt appreciated and the seniors enjoyed the young energy.

SAFETY

Resident safety is always a concern. Living spaces are designed to reduce fall risk and to enhance lighting and minimize excessive bending or reaching. Emergency response services are given code accesses to gated or secured communities. Emergency call systems are set up with directions on how to use them appropriately. If it is a fire alarm, then maps are posted to guide residents toward safe building exits and a specific outside location. The administrative office keeps records of all residents and prioritizes them for assistance in exiting the building should they need assistance with mobility equipment.

There are clear guidelines in the resident's contract that suggest when it is appropriate to consider additional assistance during illness or decline in health status. It is not unusual for seniors to insist on independence (pride or thrift) even after they begin to lose the ability to perform all activities of daily living in a safe manner. It is for the resident's safety that guidelines are set in place to ensure that they do have appropriate supervision.

STAFF MEMBERS

Many independent-living residences are part of a greater complex of living options. This type of retirement community gives people the ability to shift to other levels of living as health status changes. Some communities include independent living, residential care, and memory care. Residential care and memory care are discussed separately. In some instances, there may also be an associated skilled care facility, where the highest level of care is provided. Skilled care facilities must meet additional criteria in order to be licensed to operate within each state. The number of employees and their various roles depend on the various living options available within the individual retirement communities.

STAFF MEMBERS, SCOPE OF PRACTICE, AND EDUCATION REQUIREMENTS

Staff at independent-living communities will include the necessary administrative and management staff, including various levels of assistants. Food service often includes a head chef, prep chefs, and support staff. Grounds keepers, maintenance, security, and housekeeping (laundry) provide aesthetic and essential services.

HEALTH NURSE

Several levels of staff are available to address health concerns and to provide personal care. Some communities are large enough to provide a health nurse and personal care department separate from the residential or skilled care units. The health nurse is usually a registered nurse (RN) with an unencumbered license to practice within the state. This health nurse usually does not provide direct care (which minimizes liability insurance for the business), but serves to assess need and to act as a liaison for the resident. Education expectations (associate, bachelor's, or master's degree) for the RN may vary according to the management of the community. Usually, experience working with the geriatric population is desirable in addition to supervisory or management experience. As the need for living options for the aging population increases, specialties in geriatric, memory care, and health management options are on the upsurge as well (Capezuti et al., 2012; Kreimer, 2010).

PERSONAL CARE ASSISTANT VERSUS CERTIFIED NURSING ASSISTANT

If some home assistance is needed, scheduled visits by one of the personal care assistants can be arranged. This extra service is a separate expense from the usual monthly payment. The personal care assistant role is an entry-level position; some employers may only require a high school diploma. Often the pay is the minimum wage with little opportunity for advancement. Employers may provide on-the-job training, which is often the task protocol without the supporting science behind best practice. Each state board of nursing has specific criteria for curricula used in an approved certified nursing assistant (CNA) training program. If an applicant has completed a standardized training course and passed the state test to be a CNA, it is to the employer's advantage, but the course work and certification might make no difference in the pay scale, as the agency does not require that training.

FUNDING

Many people believe that Medicare will help to pay for living accommodations in senior care facilities. This is not true for independent-living options. Some people carry long-term insurance with home care benefits and may be able to tap that option for part of their expenses. Otherwise, most people must cover the expense by using pension, savings, and liquidation of properties (American Elder Care Research Organization [AECRO], 2014).

Costs associated with independent living may vary greatly from state to state and even within the same communities. According to the AECRO in 2014 "in the United States, the average monthly cost of independent living ranges from about $1,500 to $3,500." This expense does not cover medical bills, transportation, groceries, clothing, and other personal expenses. Making the choice to move into an independent-living setting cannot be a snap decision, but takes preplanning and perhaps the professional advice of financial advisors.

LICENSURE/REGULATORY AGENCIES

Many states do not require special licensure for independent-living communities, because the residents purchase the house, condominium, or apartment as proprietors subject to the same responsibilities and liabilities as living independently outside of the structured retirement community.

Incorporated living centers are established in many states, with more to come. One resource for this information was provided by a representative of one incorporated community that currently operates blended retirement communities in Alberta, Canada, and eight states: Washington, Oregon, Idaho, Montana, North Dakota, South Dakota, Minnesota, and Oklahoma. None of these states currently requires a special licensure or certification for the independent-living residences (Neil, 2014).

SUMMARY

- Independent residences are owned by the individual client, but the client does share in the amenities of the incorporated community.
- Residents are responsible for their own health and medical care.
- If there is physical or mental decline in a resident, it is the responsibility of that individual and/or family to arrange for additional in-home support services.
- RNs who work for a retirement community usually work in a supervisory role. They very often do not do hands-on care of any type, but may help to obtain physician orders for home health or hospice services if the need for skilled medical care occurs.
- Blended retirement communities often train their own personal care assistants, on the job, and make no pay differential for employees who have completed a standardized training program for being a CNA.
- Medicare does not help to pay for independent-living senior housing.

RESOURCES

AARP

http://assets.aarp.org/www.aarp.org_/promotions/sem/member01.html?keycode=U6TPM1&packageid=& componentid=&whocalled=promo_enroll&cmp=IVS-KNC-ACQ-PMD-ACQJOIN

Search Terms
- Advocacy information
- Local chapters
- Community services
- Valuable information for living well
- Benefits and discounts

Alliance for Retired Americans

http://retiredamericans.org

Search Terms
- State by state
- Preserve social security
- Advocate for veteran's benefits

Help Guide Organization

http://www.helpguide.org/elder/independent_living_seniors_retirement.htm

Search Terms
- Other names for independent living
- Low-income or subsidized senior housing
- Continuing care retirement community (CCRC)
- FAQ (frequently asked questions)
- Myths

Paying for Senior Care

http://www.payingforseniorcare.com/longtermcare/costs.html

Search Terms
- Help planning for care
- Paying for senior care
- Misperceptions
- FAQ
- Eldercare financial assistance locator tool

Thinking of Retiring?

http://www.socialsecurity.gov/osss/rel_1_1/pdf/en/55-plus-insert.pdf

Search Terms
- Medicare
- Monthly benefit
- Retirement age considerations

U.S. Office of Personal Management for Federal and Tribal Employees

http://www.opm.gov/about-us

Search Terms
- Life events
- Affordable Care Act
- Changes in health
- Benefits
- Retirement

REFERENCES

American Elder Care Research Organization (AECRO). (2014). *Paying for senior care*. Retrieved March 11, 2014, from http://www.payingforseniorcare.com/longtermcare/costs.html

Capezuti, E., Boltz, M., Cline, D., Dickson, V. V., Rosenberg, M. C., Wagner, L.,...Nigolian, C. (2012). Nurses improving care for health system elders—a model for optimizing the geriatric nursing practice environment. *Journal of Clinical Nursing, 21*(21–22), 3117–3125. doi: 10.1111/j.1365-2702.2012.04259.x

Howell, J. (2014). *Independent living*. Moseo Corporation-SeniorHomes.com. Retrieved March 4, 2014, from http://www.seniorhomes.com/p/independent-living

Kreimer, S. (2010). *The growing need for geriatric nurses and aging expertise across specialties*. Nursezone. Retrieved March 11, 2014, from http://www.nursezone.com/Nursing-News-Events/more-features/The-Growing-Need-forGeriatric-Nurses-and-Aging-Expertise-Across-Specialties_34380.aspx

Neil, S. D. (2014, March 12). *What licensure or certification is required to operate a blended retirement community of independent living, residential care and memory care?* Resource Assistant Manager/RCF Administrator at SDN@touchmark.com

Robinson, L., Saisan, J., & White, M. (2014). *Independent living for seniors. Helpguide.org: A trusted non-profit resource*. Retrieved March 11, 2014, from www.helpguide.org/elder/independent_living_seniors_retirement.htm

12

Assisted Living

Brenda L. Bonham Howe

WHAT IS ASSISTED LIVING?

Assisted-living facilities (ALFs) are also known as residential care facilities (RCFs) for the elderly (RCFE). Assisted-living (residential care) communities provide housing, usually in the form of an apartment or condominium. The intention of this style of assisted housing is to support a lifestyle that is as independent as possible for individuals who can no longer live alone for various reasons. These facilities are not considered medical and are not licensed to provide skilled medical care. Medical monitoring and first-aid assessment is available 24/7 with additional support assistance defined by individual need. Housing and services may be private or semiprivate.

A resident may live alone or share the apartment with a spouse or partner. Sometimes an elderly parent, who needs minimal assistance, may share the residence with another family member or close friend who also requires assistance with some aspect of activities of daily living (ADL). Sharing an apartment is one way to reduce expenses and to maintain an established companionship.

Each state has guidelines as to when the terms "assisted living," "residential care," or "bed and board" facilities are used. Many states classify senior residential options according to capacity. For instance, in California, an RCFE contains 16 or more units and the residents are 60 years of age and older (California Advocate for Nursing Home Reform [CANHR], 2014). Units may be set up as a bedroom with en suite bathroom, or a studio apartment, and sometimes as a one- or two-bedroom apartment with a kitchenette. Oregon defines ALFs as housing and supportive services for six or more residents (Oregon Department of Human Services [ODHS], 2014). The following originates from the Office of the Maine Attorney General (OMAG, 2011), which identifies are four types of RCFs.

- Level I RCF means a facility with a licensed capacity of one to two residents.
- Level II RCF means a facility with a licensed capacity of three to six residents.
- Level III RCF means a facility with a licensed capacity of three to six residents and that employs three or more persons who are not owners and are not related to the owner.
- Level IV RCF means a facility with a licensed capacity of 16 to 100 or more (OMAG, 2011).

When considering the type of residence to choose, it is important to investigate key terms and definitions related to the establishment.

AMENITIES

Many of the residences contain a kitchenette and small dining space, a living room, one or two bedrooms, and a private bathroom. Many boast of scenic views and may include a small balcony or enclosed patio. Commons areas are often featured and available for all residents, including shared dining and socialization areas. Additional features usually include a centralized laundry area for personal use, covered parking, hair and nail salon (private business), and facility transportation by appointment or preplanned route. Some communities also include restaurant dining, meeting spaces or multiuse rooms, a bank branch office, and a small "corner store."

ACTIVITIES

Most assisted-living communities offer a variety of activities to promote socialization and life enrichment. Monthly activity calendars provide an overview of planned transportation to churches, libraries, shopping centers, and recreational outings. Movie nights, guest speakers, musicians, and plays may be featured in communities that boast a small auditorium or conference center. An activities coordinator may also plan a variety of arts and crafts activities or social gatherings such as afternoon tea with cheese and fruit tasting. Sometimes, individual residents may coordinate small group activities such as Bible study, card games, and needlework clubs.

When choosing an RCF or ALF, it is good to inquire what type of budget is available to support the advertised activities.

SAFETY

Safety for the residents and staff is always a concern for any assisted-living community. The terms assisted living and residential care imply that residents have some level of physical and/or mental challenges that put them at risk of falls. Mobility issues would slow or prohibit them from exiting the building quickly in case of fire or other emergency. Every facility will have written safety procedures for resident and employee review.

One way the safety of residents is addressed is through planning of the architectural and interior design. Main entrances are wide and on ground level. All walking areas are free of obstructions and are wide enough to accommodate electrical mobility devices, wheelchairs, and walkers. Most halls will have assist rails along each side. Elevators are placed in convenient locations if the building is multistoried. Stairwells are well lit and include sturdy handrails. Living quarters include wide doorways and handicap accessible bathrooms (handrail, higher toilet, knee space under sink, and roll-in shower). Kitchenettes are well lit with storage areas placed as conveniently as possible for residents with visual and musculoskeletal limitations (American Society of Interior Designers [ASID], 2012).

Because the residents may have partial debility, the facility will have some type of call system for the individual. Bathrooms usually have a call cord or switch. Individuals may wear either a pendant or wristband that has a two-way communication feature. The resident has the option of pushing on the pendant with the message going to a personal care assistant's (PCA) cell phone or walkie-talkie. The PCA may then talk to the resident via that system to clarify what is needed. If personal help is needed, then the PCA may help or call on a staff member working closer to that resident.

STAFF MEMBERS

The staff is determined by the makeup and size of the facility. Some assisted-living communities share a campus with additional wings or separate buildings that serve the needs of people requiring skilled care or memory care. Staff resources may then be cross-trained to work in those varied settings. Some facilities may house one resident while some provide care for hundreds. The size of the facility is not a determining factor in the quality of care provided. That is one reason why it is very helpful to research facility options, and gather information about the staff at each facility and the credentials of that staff (Assisted Living Facilities Organization [ALFO], 2014b).

Before an individual or family chooses a facility, it is good to know if the facility recruits and hires staff who have trained in a standardized program recognized by the state board of nursing or if it provides onsite training. If the facility is only licensed to provide assisted living or residential care, then it is not required to hire trained nurses or caregivers who are certified as nursing assistants. If the facility also has a unit that has a special license for skilled care, then it must hire nurses and certified caregivers for that unit.

It is also helpful to ask how long the current staff has been with the facility (gives some idea of staff turnover). Taking a tour is a great way to observe how staff and residents interact as well as to note how many staff members are actually seen. Because these residential communities are not considered medical facilities, most state protocols do not require the presence of a registered nurse (RN). However, there may often be one present who serves in a primarily administrative or management capacity. Typical roles might be administrator and administrative assistant.

Other staff members/positions include:

- A medical director, who may also be an RN (in charge of health care strategies or wellness services)
- Admissions coordinator, who may be an administrative assistant, residential care manager, RN, licensed practical nurse (LPN)/licensed vocational nurse (LVN); this function may be or part of an administrative nurse's other management duties
- Director of nursing, which also may be combined with other duties as previously listed
- Staffing coordinator is a role assigned to one individual in several departments: resident assistants, custodial staff, housekeeping services, grounds keepers, kitchen and dining staff, and volunteers
- PCAs, certified nursing assistants (CNAs), LPN, and LVN roles will depend on each facility and its hiring guidelines
- A medication aide might be certified through the state after completing a standard training program. However, because many facilities are not considered medical venues, a medication aide may be an individual trained for that specific duty. It is the responsibility of management to have written protocol

for medication distribution, in addition to safety compliance guidelines. If controlled medications are ordered for a resident, then oversight by a licensed health care professional is usually required (each state has specific rules).

STAFFING REQUIREMENTS

There are state regulations that require preemployment screens, one of which is a criminal background check (this usually requires fingerprinting). Other requirements may vary by state and also the size and licenses held by the facility. The following list includes minimal requirements for the state of Florida's ALFs or RCFs, which probably stand true for most states.

- Must be 21 years of age to hold an administrative position
- Must have a high school diploma or GED
- Complete criminal background check must be conducted
- Must have successfully completed and passed the ALF core training program (Florida Agency for Health Care Administration [AHCA], 2011)
- Proof of certification or licensure is required for individuals who apply for the positions of CNA, LPN, RN, recreation therapist, or other specialty roles
- Most will also request immunization records, particularly for tuberculosis (TB) and hepatitis B. If the TB test (or recent chest x-ray) is not available, most states require the employer to provide those immunizations for the employee. The same is true for the hepatitis series.

TRAINING

In addition to any certification or licensure training that new employees possess, they must also attend new employee orientation at every facility. Each state has a list of mandatory training, which centers on safety at several levels: fire, electrical, chemical, ergonomics, and workplace violence, to name a few.

Individuals who will work directly with residents, especially those who have physical or mental impairments, must receive training on professional behavior and communication and the expectations of the facility. Protocols should be reviewed for the tasks that support ADL: assist with transfers, dressing, bathing, denture care, skin care, and so on.

If the facility has a unit dedicated to skilled care, then the RN, LPN/LVN, and CNA staff may be required to report a set number of continuing education credits to the State Board of Nursing each year. The facility is not obligated to provide those credits, but some may allow an annual education stipend for their employees.

STAFF-TO-RESIDENT RATIO

The Assisted Living Federation of America (ALFA) leaves the issue of staffing flexible so that each facility may decide what is best for its residents and resident-focused programs (Hayes, 2014). In theory, the assisted-living communities need to hire staff in sufficient numbers to adequately meet the individual needs of the residents. Within every resident population, the number of needs and degree of support needed can vary greatly. Some facilities utilize an acuity score to determine staff-to-resident ratio. This approach to staffing may become more favored as the residents age and require more assistance with ADL (Hayes, 2014).

The assisted-living community must have sufficient staff to maintain safety, order, cleanliness, and delivery of medications in a timely manner. The residents must receive the type and amount of supervision and care to meet basic needs. Depending upon the size of the facility, the night shift–staff guidelines may vary. In a very small facility, the requirement may be that a staff member is immediately available. Very often there is a sleeping area provided in very small facilities. In a larger facility, the night staff member is usually required to be immediately available and awake through the night (Texas Department of Aging and Disability Services [DADS], 2011). Many people may be surprised at the number of PCAs on duty. There might be 40 residents and 2 PCAs, 1 PCA per floor or wing. What must be considered is the acuity of the residents, as many may still be very independent and may require minimal assistance. It is important for PCAs to report decline in a resident's status in addition to increased time spent with the person. This is how the staffing coordinator knows when to make adjustments in staff-to-resident ratio.

LICENSURE/REGULATORY AGENCIES

It is important to remember that ALFs or RCFs are not considered medical facilities; therefore, they are not regulated as vigorously as facilities where skilled medical care is provided. Each state determines the standards for assisted-living residences (no federal standard exists at this time). Although individual states are moving toward defining their ALFs, there is no standard for the terms used from state to state. The terms assisted living, residential care, or personal care homes may be used to denote varied population groups. It is important to know how those terms are applied in the state where you work. It is also important to know that some licensed ALFs may also have residents with special needs (mentally challenged or dementia) even though the communities are designed for senior care (ALFO, 2014a).

Licensure for residential care or ALFs is given by each state, usually through the Department of Human Services and Seniors and People with Disabilities, community-based care. Inspection and regulatory oversight is done by the community-based care surveyors. Regulatory oversight for the license is done by the state because most of these facilities do not participate in a federal program, such as Medicare (Neil, 2014).

FUNDING

Medicare does not pay for long-term care. If a senior is hospitalized and requires rehabilitation before going back to the home setting, Medicare will pay for about 10 days in a rehabilitation facility. If the individual does not make adequate recovery to safely return home after that time period, then additional services become private pay. If the individual has long-term care insurance, that is an advantage. In order to qualify for Medicaid payment the individual must have less than $2,000 in assets. Not all facilities are Medicaid certified, therefore a transfer to another venue may be necessary. Choices may be limited as many facilities have long wait lists.

SUMMARY

- ALFs and RCFs are not licensed as medical care facilities. There may be a skilled care service on the same campus, but it will be licensed separately.
- The cost is usually determined by a basic residence fee with additional service costs determined by the need of the individual. Residences may vary in size.
- Residents are encouraged to remain as independent as possible while not compromising their safety. They may be able to manage their own medications and medical appointments. Some still have the ability to drive their own cars.
- If there is physical or mental decline in a resident, it is the responsibility of the facility staff to report changes to the family or health care representative. Each facility will have a protocol to follow in regard to contacting the resident's health care provider or emergency medical response.
- RNs who work for a retirement community usually work in an administrative capacity. They very often do not perform hands-on care of any type, but may be involved in teaching

staff, monitoring medication management, providing admission assessments, among others.
- Skilled medical services may be arranged through the physician and a home health agency.
- Blended retirement communities often train their own PCAs on the job and may make no pay differential for employees who have completed a standardized training program as CNAs.
- Medicare does not pay for long-term residential care. Payment is most often made by the individual, family, or through a long-term care insurance plan. Many individuals liquidate personal real estate and stocks to support them through their retirement years.

RESOURCES

Assisted Living Federation of America

http://www.alfa.org/alfa/default.asp

Search Terms
- News center
- Public policy
- Senior living options

California Advocates for Nursing Home Reform

http://www.canhr.org/RCFE

Search Terms
- Locate facilities
- Payment
- How to evaluate the services
- Dementia care options
- Consumer fact sheets
- Lesbian, gay, bisexual, or transgender (LGBT) issues
- Elder abuse

Move Seniors

http://www.moveseniors.com

Search Terms
- Home transition
- Find a senior specialist
- Resource center
- Types of senior relocation professionals
- Certified providers

Oregon State Department of Human Services

http://www.oregon.gov/DHS/spwpd/pages/ltc/ltc_guide/whataremy-choices.aspx

Retired Americans

www.retiredamericans.org

Search Terms
- State by state
- Newsroom
- Issues
- Preserve social security
- Advocate for veteran's benefits

Today's Caregiver

http://www.caregiver.com/articles/print/assisted_living.htm

Search Term
- Assisted-living communities checklist

Veterans Affairs

http://benefits.va.gov/atoz

Search Terms
- Adaptive equipment
- Adaptive housing
- Benefits A to Z
- Regional offices

REFERENCES

American Society of Interior Designers (ASID). (2012). *Design for active aging.* Retrieved March 23, 2014, from http://www.asid.org/content/design-active-aging

Assisted Living Facilities Organization (ALFO). (2014a). *What is an assisted living facility?* Retrieved March 7, 2014, from http://www.assistedliving-facilities.org/blog/what-is-an-assisted-living-facility

Assisted Living Facilities Organization (ALFO). (2014b). *Assisted living facility staff.* Retrieved March 6, 2014, from on http://www.assistedlivingfacilities.org/blog/assisted-living-facility-staff

California Advocate for Nursing Home Reform (CANHR). (2014). *Residential care facilities for the elderly.* San Francisco, CA: CANHR. Retrieved September 9, 2014, from www.canhr.org

Florida State. (2011). *Minimum staffing requirements.* Department of Elder Affairs: Florida affordable assisted living. Retrieved March 11, 2014, from http://elderaffairs.state.fl.us/faal/operator/minimum.html

Hayes, N. (2014). *Q&A. Caring.com: Online resource for caregivers.* Retrieved March 23, 2014, from http://www.caring.com/questions/caregivers-to-residents-ratios-in-assisted-living

Neil, S. D. (2014, March 12). *What licensure or certification is required to operate a blended retirement community of independent living, residential care and memory care?* Resource Assistant Manager/RCF Administrator at SDN@touchmark.com

Office of the Maine Attorney General (OMAG). (2011). *Regulations governing the licensing and functioning of assisted house programs: Assisted living programs.* Maine Department of Health & Human Services. Retrieved September 9, 2014, from www.maine.gov/dhhs/oads/aging/long-term/residential-careshtml

Oregon Department of Human Services (ODHS). (2014). *Definition of assisted living facility. Oregon administrative rules* (Ch. 411). Retrieved September 9, 2014, from www.dhs.state.or.us/policy/spd/rules/411_054\pdf

Texas Department of Aging and Disability Services (DADS). (2011). *Licensing standards for assisted living facilities.* Retrieved March 20, 2014, from http://texasagingnetwork.com/assisted-living/assisted-living-staffing-requirements.htm

U.S. Department of Labor. (2012). *Tuberculosis testing. Occupational safety and health administration.* Retrieved March 24, 2014, from https://www.osha.gov/SLTC/tuberculosis/index.html

13

Long-Term Care

Kaye Conrath

WHAT IS LONG-TERM CARE?

Long-term care (LTC) facilities are typically geriatric caregiving facilities, although clients of any age may be found within. Katz, Karuza, Intrator, and Mor (2009) reported 1.6 million residents in LTC, which will double by the year 2030 (p. 3). Although other housing options are increasingly available, LTC facilities are a major resource in the health care continuum in the United States, because they accommodate increasingly frail residents whose hospital stays have been dramatically shortened (Katz et al., 2009, p. 5).

Care within the facilities is delineated as either custodial care or skilled care. Clients within either category are cared for, but the source of payment may vary based on the level of care needed. Custodial care is provided to assist clients with activities of daily living (ADL). These are activities a person completes on a typical day and include dressing, eating, bed mobility, toileting, and transferring. Payment sources for this level of care can include private pay, Medicaid, Veterans Affairs, and/or a privately funded LTC insurance policy. Conversely, skilled care includes interventions, such as rehabilitation therapies and IV infusions, that require the skill of a trained professional (Centers for Medicare and Medicaid Services [CMS], 2014). These are activities that require the skills and services of medical professionals such as nurses, physical therapists (PTs), and speech therapists (STs).

LTC facilities also provide services such as medication administration, diet and nutrition counseling and management, recreational activities, psychosocial services, discharge planning, and dementia care.

STAFF MEMBERS, SCOPE OF PRACTICE, AND EDUCATION REQUIREMENTS

Staffing at nursing facilities includes the necessary administrative staff, custodial staff, and food service staff.

At a minimum there must be a registered nurse (RN) scheduled for 8 hours of work every day. RNs have the broadest scope of practice, although it might vary from state to state. RNs are able to administer medications, complete wound care, manage ventilators, act as a case manager, assist with patient education, and actively participate in discharge planning. These RNs conduct patient assessments and confer with the physician to process verbal or written directions from those physicians in order to efficiently implement changes in care orders. Educational programs can be as short as 2 years for associate degree nurses (ADNs), 4 years for baccalaureate degree nurses (BSNs), and 6 years for master's prepared nurses (MSNs).

Federal regulations also require a licensed practical nurse (LPN), licensed vocational nurse (LVN), or an RN to be scheduled to work the rest of the day. The educational programs for the LPN or LVN are generally 18 months, with most programs embedded within a community college.

Certified nursing assistants (CNA), commonly referred to as "aides," are generally the largest group of employees. They may be certified and licensed as such, or they may be in the process of completing their certification program and acting as a nursing assistant registered (NAR). In either capacity, these are the primary caregivers that are generally responsible for helping clients with bathing, dressing, eating, mobility, and other routine ADL. Depending upon varying state laws, these caregivers have limited ability to help beyond the custodial activities listed.

Each facility employs additional professional staff to meet diverse client needs. These staff members include social workers, dieticians, and therapists. Social workers help deal with personal and social concerns and are often very involved in discharge planning. Dieticians are either on staff or contracted by the facility to help provide evaluation and treatment options for clients with nutritional problems or concerns. Physical rehabilitation may be done by therapists employed or contracted by the facility. These include PTs, occupational therapists (OTs), recreational therapists (RTs), and STs. Each of these therapy specialties can help clients regain losses caused by injury or disease and can play a key role in helping clients return to their prior level of functioning. Certification programs are available to allow therapy assistants that have not completed the entire educational program to assist in rehabilitation activities.

When discussing the health care team and services, we must not forget the physician (MD) or other medical providers such as a physician's assistant (PA) and/or nurse practitioner (NP). These professionals coordinate with the facility to provide medical care, although they are not necessarily a staff member of the facility. Ideally, the provider would visit the client at the facility, although this does not happen at every facility or with every physician.

Each client needs to have a designated physician prior to admission. This physician has to agree to "follow" or care for the client, although he or she may require the client to travel to the physician's office. Often, the client will be required to see the physician at the office for routine check-ups or significant issues, with the PA or NP paying visits to the client's facility between MD visits.

FUNDING

Payment sources for this level of care typically include Medicare, Medicare supplemental policies, private insurance policies, Veterans Affairs, and even private pay.

It is very important to establish the client's care coverage prior to the actual admission in order to provide informed consent to the client and his or her family. The expense of a nursing home stay was averaged at $222/day for a semiprivate room in 2012 (MetLife, 2014). That was an average for room and board, and did not include additional services such as prescriptions, therapies, and special equipment needs.

LICENSURE/REGULATORY AGENCIES

Licensure of an LTC facility must be done at the state level at a minimum. However, in order to seek reimbursement from the government through Medicare or Medicaid programs, it must also be licensed and inspected as a federally licensed facility.

Any federally licensed facility is inspected initially and then is inspected no more than every 15 months after that. This inspection is conducted by the state agency, which has local jurisdiction. Additional inspections may be conducted on an as-needed basis to investigate isolated issues and concerns, which are either reported by the facility itself and/or by any person who has complaints against the facility.

SUMMARY

- Long-term care provides ongoing custodial or skilled care for individuals of all ages.
- Payment sources include private pay, Medicaid, the Veterans Administration, and privately funded long-term care insurance.

- Federal regulations set the standards for staff requirements in licensure, certification, and continuing education needs.
- Licensure of the facility is done at the state level.

RESOURCES

Official U.S. Government Site for Medicare Coverage

http://www.medicare.gov/coverage/nursing-home-care.html

Search Terms
- Is my test, item, or service covered?
- Find nursing homes
- Other long-term care choices

Sites Related to Long-Term Care

www.longtermcarelink.net/eldercare/long_term_care.htm

Search Terms
- What is long-term care?
- Custodial versus skilled care
- Long-term care statistics: age, length of stay...

REFERENCES

Centers for Medicare and Medicaid Services (CMS). (2013). *Nursing home compare*. Retrieved August 24, 2013, from http://www.medicare.gov/NursingHomeCompare/About/Nursing-Home-info.html

Katz, P., Karuza, J., Intrator, O., & Mor, V. (2009). Nursing home physician specialists: A response to the workforce crisis in long-term care. *Annals of Internal Medicine, 150*(6), 411–413. Retrieved March 1, 2014, from CINAHL database at Foley Center Library www.gonzaga.edu

MetLife. (2014). *Market survey of long-term care costs*. Retrieved February 17, 2014, from http://www.metlife.com/mmi/research/2012-market-survey-long-term-care-costs.html

14

Alzheimer's and Memory Care

Brenda L. Bonham Howe

RESIDENTIAL CARE TRANSFORMATION INTO MEMORY CARE

Memory care is specialized assisted living (or residential care). Licensure in most states is through the Department of Human Services (DHS). In the past, all clients with the diagnosis of dementia or Alzheimer's disease (AD) were often moved into assisted living, adult foster care homes, or skilled care in the general population of those communities (see Chapter 12 for information about assisted living).

Some of the symptoms demonstrated by memory-challenged individuals can be very disruptive and disconcerting for residents who are not so cognitively impaired. Behaviors exhibited may include restlessness, wandering into other rooms (moving things or taking things), asking repetitive questions, shouting, and lacking inhibition. Imagine a naked resident wandering into the dining room for lunch. Or, think about how irritating it may be to have someone in the commons area repeating, "Yes, Yes, Yes, Yes, Yes," in various levels of voice (from soft to shrill).

Numbers Speak for Themselves

According to the 2014 Alzheimer's Facts and Figures, one in nine older Americans has AD. There are 5.2 million Americans (of all ages) with the diagnosis of Alzheimer's. A news release from the World Health Organization (WHO) in 2012 reported that there are nearly 35.6 million people living with dementia. Dementia refers to symptoms that may be caused by myriad factors such as medication, infection, cardiovascular disease (CVD), and so on. Cases of dementia are expected to double by 2030 (65.7 million) and triple by 2050 (115.4 million).

CAREGIVER BURDEN

The cost associated with caring for people with dementia was between $160 billion and $215 billion in 2010. Costs will continue to escalate with the increasing older population. These two facts should prove to be red flags for existing and future care facilities. Corporations and investors who refuse to invest in memory care programs will face significant challenges. One reason is the growing burden on family caregivers. The second reason is the growing interest in researching facilities for aging parents. As the family members become more educated about living options for their loved ones, the more particular they will be about the type of facility they choose (Thompson, 2013).

It is true that many spouses or family members become caregivers for their memory-impaired loved one. However, caring for someone with any form of dementia may become a heavy burden. Individuals with dementia may demonstrate an array of troublesome behaviors that can be a very emotional and psychological drain on the caregiver. Many with dementia wander through the night and this disturbs the sleep of caregivers and may lead to unsafe situations as well. At some point, many caregivers realize the role is just too exhausting for them. That is when they must consider doing whatever it takes to place their loved ones in a safe environment.

MEMORY CARE HAS A NEW FACE

The philosophy of memory care has made almost a complete turnaround in the past 20 years. "Reorient the patient frequently" is part of the philosophy taught when this author went through nursing school a few decades ago. A recent clinical experience with her own nursing students in a memory care facility proved to provide an ah-ha moment of appreciation for the new face of memory care philosophy.

Maria Montessori (1870–1952)

Maria Montessori was an Italian medical doctor, pediatrician, researcher, and educator (ahead of her time in many respects). She first pursued techniques for educating children who were thought disabled. One of her goals was simply to help those individual children attain their own highest possible level of skill. Her work was proven effective enough on the developmentally disabled that she decided to move forward and try her teaching philosophy on "normal" children. In 1907, the Italian government gave her that opportunity and the first of many schools was opened. By 1925, there were 1,000 Montessori schools in the United States. Her legacy continues to this day (A&E Television Network [A&E], 2014).

The Philosophy in Memory Care

Montessori's system of education is both a philosophy of child growth and a rationale of guiding such growth. The basis is the child's developmental needs for freedom within limits, a prepared environment (controlled exposure and experiences), which stimulates intellectual, physical, and social growth. It is not unusual for people to make the observation that individuals with dementia often seem to have regressed into an early stage of development. Sometimes they appear to be a child trapped in an old body. They have lost the ability to take an active part in their environment, other than to wander and demonstrate agitation. Caregivers who are prepared to work with these individuals hope to provide activities, stimulation, and guidance to help the individuals retain their remaining abilities and perhaps decrease unsafe behavior (or the frequency of undesirable behaviors). Participation in activities is encouraged at the pace the individual is capable of traveling (Lin, Huang, Watson, Wu, & Lee, 2011).

The prepared environment is set up to promote self-directed learning. An important aspect of the environment is also the supportive environment with the teacher in a trusted position as facilitator of learning. The teacher encourages, respects, and loves each of her students. The students are appreciated as unique individuals (Montessoriway, 2014).

Client-Centered Care

How Montessori's teaching philosophy translates into memory-care settings first includes preparation of the environment. The building design first takes safety into consideration. Keypad locks are common in order to access the interior of the care unit. The code is changed occasionally to discourage any alert resident from exploring the parking lot or neighborhood.

Visually, the area is designed to simulate a comfortable home environment rather than a health care facility. The colors are warm, the area is defined in a specific home-style kitchen area and common dining room (for groups of four). There is a sitting area designed for small group presentations (a media room) and a fireplace room, which may also include a large screen television. A piano is often provided for residents or guest musicians.

The floor plan of the unit is usually in a figure eight, to provide a guided path, which helps residents to avoid becoming stuck in corners. The caregivers' work spaces are often situated to provide an overview of the commons areas. Colorful artwork lines the walls through each hall, picturing scenes likely to trigger resident memories (a horse, a dog, flowers, vegetables, fruit basket, farm house, old car, wheat fields, etc.).

Studio apartments provide a private area for each resident to have personal and familiar belongings. Family photos and personal artwork provide the potential of touching a personal comfort zone. Tactile items are also a source of comfort and many residents enjoy a stuffed animal or find comfort in a baby doll.

Teacher Caregivers

Caregivers trained to work with memory-care clients play a dual role. They are present to provide care for activities of daily living (ADL), to make sure nutritional needs are met, and to oversee medication management. As memory-care facilitators, they encourage client participation in the commons areas. Structured activities provide some direction and routine through the day. Residents take part in group and individual activities at their own pace. Each resident is seen as a unique person of value.

Many residents seem to reside in some specific memories of the past. The old concept of reorienting the individual has become "meet them where they are." Two ladies walked up to a caregiver and said, "Excuse me. We're not sure where we're supposed to be." The caregiver responded, "Oh, I'm not sure either. Let's walk down here and look at the schedule on the wall." After reviewing the schedule, they all agreed it was time to go to the media area for chair exercises. That knowledge provided immediate (if only temporary) relief for the two ladies as they headed down the hall to the media area.

Activities

A variety of activities provides numerous opportunities to draw residents into events that trigger some interest. Taking part in planned opportunities helps to stimulate cognitive abilities. Simplified books may be provided for a weekly book club. Some of the book topics include brief biographies of famous people, or tell how certain popular products were invented. The residents who are able to read are encouraged to take turns reading a page (Cline, 2006).

The media area is often the venue for large-screen slide shows. Sometimes, the topics are about current or historical events. Residents are invited to read the slides and to share any thoughts they have about the subject or the ideas. Slide shows of Americana, including patriotic songs, may be a popular activity. Lifelong learning may include topics such as the current Olympics or the migration of monarch butterflies.

SUMMARY

- Concern for care of the current and future population of aging Americans increases when considering the statistics that demonstrate a significantly increasing population diagnosed with dementia and AD.
- Research has inspired a shift in thinking about the care of individuals with memory impairment.
- Maria Montessori's philosophy of teaching has evolved from application for children to adults with cognitive changes due to factors that contribute to dementia.
- Memory-care facilities are being designed to help promote the type of environment that may enable residents to maintain the cognitive ability they retain at the time of admission.
- Ongoing education for caregivers, family members, and the community may help to ensure this proactive approach to memory care.

RESOURCES

Anderson, S. (2011). A loving approach to dementia care: Making meaningful connections with the person who has Alzheimer's disease or other dementia or memory loss. *Australasian Journal on Ageing, 30*(3), 171. doi: 10.1111/j.1741-6612.2011.00560.x

REFERENCES

A&E Television Network (A&E). (2014). *Maria Montessori*. Retrieved May 19, 2014, from www.biography.com/people/maria-montessori-9412528#educational legacy&awesm=~oELxbyhWdqwCKQ

Cline, J. (2006). Montessori-based dementia care. *Kansas Nurse, 81*(9), 14. ISSN: 0022–8710. Retrieved May 19, 2014, from http://web.b.ebscohost.com.proxy.foley.gonzaga.edu/ehost/detail?vid=7&sid=6c1cd110-6e0b-4eb9-9b06 3af77b8d7d51%40sessionmgr112&hid=123&bdata= JnNpdG U9ZWhvc3QtbGl2ZQ%3d%3d#db=rzh&AN=2009351813.

Lin, L.-C., Huang, Y.-J., Watson, R., Wu, S.-C., & Lee, Y.-C. (2011). Using a Montessori method to increase eating ability for institutionalised residents with dementia: A crossover design. *Journal of Clinical Nursing, 20*(21/22), 3092–3101. ISSN: 0962–1067. Retrieved May 19, 2014, from http://proxy.foley.gonzaga.edu/login?url=http://search.ebscohost.com/login.aspx?direct=true&db=rzh&AN=2011304875&site=ehost-live

Montessoriway. (2014). *Montessori philosophy*. Retrieved May 19, 2014, from http://montessoriway.org/index.html

Thompson, J. (2013). Rethinking memory care. *Long Term Living, 92*(6), 38–41. Resource guide retrieved May 19, 2014, from http://web.a.ebscohost.com.proxy.foley.gonzaga.edu/ehost/detail?sid=c52a847e-3d4e-42ca-a6d6-1c6d327641ae%40sessionmgr4003&vid=6&hid=4101&bdata=JnN pdGU9ZWhvc3 QtbGl2ZQ%3d%3d#db=rzh&AN=2012256186.

World Health Organization (WHO). (2012). *Dementia cases set to triple by 2050 but still largely ignored*. Retrieved May 19, 2014, from www.who.int/mediacentre/news/releases/2012/dementia_20120411/en

15

Additional Community Health Resources for the Financially Compromised

Brenda L. Bonham Howe

Sometimes there is no easy one-step solution to making helpful connections for a client. It requires someone with patience and perseverance, much like a detective on a trail that is sometimes vague and fraught with irritants and obstacles. After making an inquiry to a local hospital discharge planner Katie Kimmel (personal communication, April 12, 2014; Local Parish Nurse Association Meetings, Bend, OR), the author learned that one must simply make a list and start making phone calls. There are so many variables (current funding, protocol, staffing, etc.) involved that the resource available this week may not be available the next week.

Kimmel (personal communication, April 12, 2014) recommends the use of the nursing process: assessment, planning, intervention, and evaluation. First, identify the needs of the client. List potential community resources. The contact list may be given to the client. It may be necessary or appropriate to make contacts for the client, but Kimmel suggests being "the guide and motivator, not the driver."

Teach the client the art of resourcing to empower him or her to take the next step as independently as possible.

WHERE TO START

A phone book or Internet access may be the first necessary tool to find local service agencies, both government and private. Organize resource information and store it for easy future reference. There may be many resources in the local community, and sometimes they form coalitions of similar means in order to avoid duplication of services with the hope of assisting more people.

Local resources often include community and senior centers, council on aging, homeless outreach, cultural resources, faith outreach, educational resources, and support groups for specific health challenges. Sometimes several outreach organizations fund publication of a resource guide for seniors. The local senior center or Department of Human Services is often the distribution point for the publication. Individuals may choose to create a customized resource list that will usually include the following: name of the organization, contact person, phone number, e-mail address, location, and specific services offered.

Community Health Clinics

The names of community health clinics may vary from state to state, but the service goals are the same. They exist to serve the primary health care needs of more than 22 million patients in more than 9,000 locations across America. They play a vital role in America's health care system, providing low-cost health services for millions of uninsured, working poor, and newly jobless Americans (National Association of Community Health Centers [NACHC], 2014).

Parish Nurses

Parish nurses have made a gradual comeback, but may be a new concept to many. A parish nurse is a registered nurse (RN) who serves a church or parish in a volunteer or paid position. The name "parish" originally meant the whole neighborhood and included the congregation as well as the surrounding neighborhood. The Reverend Dr. Granger Westberg began parish nursing in the mid-1980s in Chicago, bringing back nursing outreach as done by religious orders in Europe and America in the 1800s. He provided a vital link between health systems and congregations. "He urged his hospital to launch a program in area congregations to provide 'parish nurses' who would reach out into the community to build bridges of healing and hope" (QueensCare, 2014).

Parish nurses are the resource persons in the congregation. They are health advisors, educators, advocates, liaisons to faith and community resources, and volunteers, and work closely with the pastor and congregation to provide the necessary resources. Parish nurses may be found in service for Christian churches, Muslim mosques, and Jewish synagogues (International Parish Nurse Resource Center [IPNRC], 2014).

"WHO DO I CALL FIRST?"

Who is called first will depend on the client's immediate need and the current location. Nurses are taught and encouraged to develop critical-thinking skills. We are not expected to solve everyone else's problems, though we would love to possess that power. Our referrals will also depend on the need of the client.

If a nurse is in his or her work setting, it is important to know what the employer policies are in place for referring clients to community resources. Some agencies may have specific persons assigned that task, such as discharge planners or medical social workers.

When finances are extremely compromised, most health care facilities have someone in the business office who will work with the client to try and establish a payment plan. For any debt, it is far better to contact the company and explain the situation rather than ignore the notices. Even making minimal payments demonstrates the desire to acknowledge and pay off the debt. See the Resources section for access to state-by-state links to potential financial assistance programs.

SUMMARY

- There is no set pattern for referring clients to community health resources.
- The referral depends upon the need of the client.
- There are many potential resources, both local and national.
- It is helpful to know what resources or lists are available in the facility or agency where the client is seen.
- Sometimes it takes the work of a detective to assist and empower clients to move toward helpful resources.

RESOURCES

AARP

www.aarp.org

Search Terms
- In your state
- Benefits
- Discounts
- Coupons
- Diversity

American Red Cross

www.americanredcross.org

Search Terms
- Find your local chapter
- Get assistance—disaster relief

Easter Seals Senior Community Service Employment Program

www.EasterSeals.com

Search Terms
- Senior services
- Day services
- Medical rehabilitation
- Services for caregivers

Independent Living Resources

www.ilr.org

Search Terms
- Services
- Programs
- Partnerships

National Patient Advocate Foundation

www.npaf.org

Search Terms
- Federal
- State
- Resources for advocacy

Need Help Paying Bills?

http://www.needhelppayingbills.com/html/about_us.html

Search Terms
- State and local programs
- Rent help
- Electric and heating bills
- Debt counseling
- Medical bills and free health
- Charity assistance
- Mortgage help
- Other debts
- Low interest loans

REFERENCES

International Parish Nurse Resource Center (IPNRC). (2014). *Church health center*. Retrieved May 26, 2014, from www.parishnurses.org

National Association of Community Health Centers (NACHC). (2014). *About our health centers*. Retrieved May 26, 2014, from http://www.nachc.com/about-our-health-centers.cfm

QueensCare. (2014). *Parish nursing fact sheet*. Retrieved May 26, 2014, from http://www.queenscare.org/files/qc/pdfs/ParishNursingFactSheet0311.pdf

16

Why Must Clients and Caregivers Embrace Self-Advocacy?

Brenda L. Bonham Howe and Esther Freeman

Clients and caregivers need to become their own advocates, because all health care workers, medical clinics, and facilities are not created equal. However, many people believe that the term "health or healthy" indicates something that is good for them. In the American culture, people are bombarded by commercials and programs about beneficial health products. Actual employees of various types of home care services offer sincere concern and have potential clients' best interests at heart, which is why that particular service should be called for assistance. No doubt there is some truth to what is advertised, but there is something to be gained by the marketers and it is always about profit. After all, the most generous not-for-profit agency must make enough money to stay in business.

There are still individuals in every community who believe "the doctor knows everything about me," or "the doctor is always right," or "oh, I let the doctor keep track of that information for me." The author, who once worked in a phone triage role, had many callers make those statements, in addition to, "I can't remember what I'm allergic to, but the doctor knows." The last comment is an excellent example of an individual not taking personal responsibility for knowledge that may be life threatening in an emergency situation. It also seems rather egocentric, because why would the doctor be expected to remember every client's medications or allergies?

HUMAN SIDE OF PROFESSIONALS

Professional health care providers are human, too. They are susceptible to fatigue, illness, mental health issues, forgetfulness, and mistakes. Doctors and nurses do not set out to intentionally harm other people, but statistics prove that this happens on a daily basis (Bonnifield & Cohen, 2014). Being familiar with the primary caregiver is more important than ever, because individuals are seen by so many specialists. Forming a partner type of relationship with the primary health care providers will reduce the potential for error.

Seeing multiple health care providers really complicates accurate and effective communication. It is a wonderful process for miscommunication unless someone takes control and acts as the communication moderator. Who will do that unless it is the client or a designated caregiver (case manager, family member, etc.)? Medical office staff will usually try to assist, but they work in a high-stress, fast-paced setting, and they may not have time to simply dedicate to a client's communication dilemma.

TAKE CHARGE OF MEDICAL RECORDS

The primary health care provider must always be kept in the communication loop. Specialists will send a copy of visit notes and reports from studies or labs. However, that information may disappear into the cosmic reaches of the fax machine, or be accidentally filed in someone else's chart. How is a client to cope with the inconvenient truths of nondelivery and misfiling? The answer is, take control and ask for copies of everything to be sent directly to the client or caregiver (case manager, family member), and file it where it could be readily found. Take the information to the next appointment with the primary care provider to make sure they have copies (see Appendix 16A at the end of this chapter for a discussion of a personal medical notebook).

DOCTOR DEFICIT

The United States has a shortage of primary health care providers, especially in rural settings (Health Resources and Services Administration [HRSA], 2014). The providers barely have time to address the immediate care needs of clients. Appointment time slots have become shorter over the years as providers try to see more clients in order to maintain the annual financial goal. Individual clients and caregivers need to buy into the concept that they are responsible for proactive participation in their own health care concerns. "Most doctors go into health care with an overwhelming desire to help people. Providing care is a two-way street between a doctor and patient. Working together, they get the best results" (Cosgrove, 2013; see Appendix 16A).

IDEAL IS NOT REALITY

Federal and state health care standards reflect the ideal of best practice and equal delivery to every population group in the United States. Licensing agencies publish handbooks and manuals of regulatory standards for every health care facility and agency in order to continue serving the community. Medical and nursing students are taught the best practice standards, because best practice ensures quality outcomes.

Who provides the oversight for best practices and how often are they able to do so? Inspectors may be scheduled annually or every

2 years, depending on the specific agency. Surprise inspections may occur at random or as a follow-up due to complaints filed by clients or family members. Just how thorough those inspections may be also depends on how the protocol is written. If a door is closed or locked, is the inspector allowed to request going into that space? How many hours are allowed for inspection? After all, the inspectors are paid for their work and their employer is conscious of keeping the payroll at a minimum. The inspector may be scheduled for more than one facility per workday. Time is money and money is time—a forever concern for the bottom line. If the inspectors cannot guarantee that residents are receiving best practice care, who can?

"THE NURSE"

What happened to "Wonder Nurse" or those "angels in white caps"? Sorry to say, they are urban legends based on partial truth and imaginative embellishment by adoring clients and Hollywood. The nursing shortage is a well-publicized concern. Although many nurses, especially new graduates, are looking for employment opportunities, for too many years work in geriatric residential settings has not been viewed as one of the more prestigious nursing roles. However, gerontology nursing is one of the rapidly emerging specialty areas for nurses. With that being said, is "the nurse" the person who can guarantee that residents receive best practice quality care?

Clients and caregivers must understand that many facilities are not required to retain a registered nurse (RN) as a staff member. In other facilities, the RN may work primarily in an administrative role with limited one-on-one time for residents. This information is also discussed in the chapters about long-term care, residential care, and skilled care facilities. The RN often has supervisory responsibilities for direct-care staff providers, but how can that nurse ensure that the care plan tasks are actually performed? Although the nurse may possess good work ethics, her workload may prevent her from checking on clients often enough to confirm that caregivers are fulfilling their assigned duties.

Family members or a personal case manager may make unannounced, short visits at various times through the week. They need to make sure that the resident is clean: Is hair combed, face washed, hands cleaned, food stuck in the teeth, and so on? Assist the resident to the bathroom and allow some amount of privacy; check the brief for soiling; check the skin for dried stool, urine odor, redness, or rash; and update one of the caregivers if the brief was changed during the visit. Frequent urinary tract infections may be an indication that brief changes and good perianal care need to be performed more frequently.

STAFF RETENTION

"Caregiver turnover for senior care companies can be as high as 75%" (Northcutt, 2011). Turnover costs companies many thousands of dollars a year in the hiring and training process. RNs are part of the turnover cycle, but at a lower percentile than resident care assistants and certified nursing assistants.

Why is the turnover so high? Of course, some turnover can be attributed to low census, but more often caregivers, particularly patient care assistants or certified nursing assistants, report issues like working a high client-to-staff ratio, too much heavy lifting, muscle strain or injury, fluctuating work schedules, difficult clients or coworkers, low pay, and inflexible staffing (no one to cover for special day off requests), or lack of training and support. Most of all, it's very hard work—physically and emotionally draining work.

Earlier chapters discussed the fact that some caregivers are trained on the job and others attend a training program approved by the state board of nursing. Standard or on-the-job training does not ensure that each person will complete the training with personal high moral and ethical standards though an effort is made to teach them. Time and work experience may contribute to wear and tear on the person's outlook on work and that often results in poor-quality performance.

MORAL AND ETHICAL BURNOUT

"In 1984, Andrew Jameton defined 'moral distress' as a phenomenon in which one knows the right action to take, but is constrained from taking it" (Epstein & Delgado, 2010). Many health care providers experience personal moral and ethical turmoil because they are not able to provide quality care to their clients. There are many reasons for this inability, but primarily it is due to an inadequate ratio of staff to clients. With the concern about soaring health care costs, some of the cutbacks have also reduced the variety and quantity of medical supplies available. This transition reflects the swing from individualized care to one-size-fits-all (dressings, products carried by the facility pharmacy supplier, etc.).

Some health services and residential facilities used to provide personal care items such as adult briefs, personal hygiene wipes, soaps, shampoos, conditioners, combs, brushes, and oral and nail care products. Now, many of those services no longer provide the items. Some provide a maximum number per month. Often, caregivers do not have the supplies they need to perform quality care and feel helpless when their employer will not order more until it is time to utilize the next disbursement of funds.

MORAL RESIDUE

Moral residue is a phenomenon described by Webster and Bayliss (2010) who said that moral residue is "that which each of us carries with us from those times in our lives when in the face of moral distress we have seriously compromised ourselves or allowed ourselves to be compromised" (Epstein & Delbado, 2010). In these situations, one's moral values have been violated due to limitations beyond one's control. These experiences create a moral wound of having had to act against one's values. Moral residue is long lasting and deeply sowed into one's thoughts and views of the self. This phase of moral distress can be damaging to the self-respect and one's career.

EMPOWERING THE INNER ADVOCATE

The *International Council of Nurses Code of Ethics 2012* states that it is part of the nurses' role to "enable patient empowerment" (Burkhardt & Nathaniel, 2008). Nurses have to demonstrate respect for others, develop a trusting relationship, and provide encouragement to improve client and caregiver self-esteem. This may be the earliest step of empowerment, but the steps are moving in the right direction. According to Burkhardt and Nathaniel (2008), Gibson describes empowerment as "a social process of recognizing, promoting, and enhancing people's abilities to meet their own needs, solve their own problems and mobilize the necessary resources…a process of helping people to assert control over the factors which affect their own health." Individual clients and caregivers must play an active role in their own health care in order to improve communication with providers, avoid errors, and have a clear understanding of contractual agreements for services. There are many online resources and books to learn more about taking care of aging relatives.

PLAN POSITIVE RELIEF

So many aspects of thinking about health care needs can be exhausting. The majority of individuals receiving live-in assistance are cared for by a family member. There are many activities that provide some rest and relaxation and at the same time may help a loved one to retain or maintain some of his or her functional and cognitive abilities.

One area to research, not discussed in earlier chapters, is therapeutic recreation. Certified recreation therapists are often employed by hospitals, mental health hospitals, long-term care centers, and parks and recreation districts. The following article provides some details and examples of activities that are beneficial for use with geriatric clients and their caregivers.

RECREATION AND RECREATION THERAPY FOR THE GERIATRIC POPULATION

Working with the geriatric population can range from community to short-term care, long-term care, and mental health settings. Each brings an important aspect to care, but the ultimate standard is that everyone deserves the access to recreation. This tenet is borne out in the Americans with Disabilities Act; its earliest predecessor known as Public Law 94–142 from 1974. Inclusion is more commonly the "buzz" word today, but earlier the terminology was mainstreaming people into recreation programs. However, for some people being included in the norm or mainstream of programs or activities cannot or will not be possible, dependent upon the level of one's disability. A stroke or brain injury that takes away use of one or more limbs may be deemed as an impossible feat to overcome, yet I have seen people surpass that hurdle and allow a return to community-living environments.

With any client the recreation therapist wishes to improve his or her functioning ability through the social, emotional, cognitive, and physical domains. Recreation programming must, therefore, be variable. Within an institutional setting only a portion of those domains may be met each day, depending on the number of clientele within the facility and the recreation staffing. It should be noted here, however, that an activity therapist who works in a nursing home setting generally is not a recreation therapist and, by activity director standards of practice, his or her depth of educational knowledge is far less than the minimum of a 4-year therapeutic recreation degree for a certified therapeutic recreation specialist (CTRS). Due to funding limitations, a great number of nursing and long-term care facilities do not hire someone who is a CTRS. Mental health hospitals today, however, do require a CTRS along with other allied professionals, including occupational therapists.

Let us look at some possible programs for our aging population. Physical exercise, also referred to as the psychomotor domain, is critical to stabilizing or even improving eye–hand coordination. Swimming is a great tool for relief of multiple sclerosis pain, improvement of amputees, and strengthening of people who have had strokes. Most nursing homes do not have swimming pools, although the veteran's hospitals usually do, and arrangements can also be made with local agencies such as Young Men's Christian Association (YMCA), hotels/motels, or parks and recreation facilities. In some communities, there is Easter Seal, which is not limited to facility usage for children. Initially, just getting into the pool may be a difficult task, but as the individual gains strength along with improved social skills after an illness, injury, or loss of physical strength, he or she may easily be referred to a local swim program. As of 2014, there are new rules for pool access established by the Americans with Disabilities Act. For some people, the transitioning into the use of swimming for exercise or improvement may require mentoring either by a volunteer followed by the recreation therapist, or by the recreation therapist himself or herself.

Swimming alone is not the goal a recreation therapist or inclusion therapist has when he or she is working with a geriatric patient. Swimming is just one of the few methods of exercise for aging or geriatric adults. Exercise of any type can be useful. In working with people who have multiple sclerosis, for example, they admit that retaining as much of their range of motion as possible is critical. Making a rotating motion at the ankles or wrists is useful for them.

A recreation therapist wants to make these types of exercise fun. There are many "sit and be fit" exercise programs both in written form and in video form. Adaptation is the key.

Lidia Garbach and Ann Pardo wrote a book called *Exercises Can Be Fun* for working in group programs for older adults. This book shares a few simple methods of starting and sustaining an exercise group or club. This writer believes, too, that using a few dance steps and music familiar to the geriatric group one is working with, and teaching the chair exercises, are a few of the adaptations that keep an individual engaged. Encouraging the participant to sing to the music or to choose a favorite exercise and perform it provides an onus of control.

Yoga is used to assist with balance and has been utilized with geriatric patients. Tai chi similarly works with balance, but caution should be exercised with both yoga and tai chi regarding the present functioning ability of all participants. Remember, in recreation therapy, anything can be adapted in order to offer inclusion of all participants.

During 1983 to 1984, this author worked in the Klamath County Nursing Home. On days when nursing staff had a few minutes to spare they were engaged by the recreation therapist in a parachute activity. The "Vienna Waltzes" were put on, people in wheelchairs and staff made a huge circle to accommodate holding the parachute, and foam balls were thrown into the center of the parachute. When the music was loud and broad, we made great waves when arms were lifted high. When the notes were rapid, we made little waves. This action brought laughter, helped open lungs for oxygen as arms were lifted, gave reminiscence through familiar music, and supplied an opportunity for social interactions. In the 1970s, there was a slogan trademarked in Australia and used in parks and recreation facilities throughout the world: "Life. Be in it." Helping the geriatric person gain even some independence and sense of value can indeed help him or her increase involvement in life (see Appendix 16B).

Cognitive activities are also critical for geriatric clientele. We all have heard from many people, even those who aren't therapists or nurses, that working on crossword puzzles and Sudoku is a good skill for keeping one's mind alert. Another good skill is completing dot-to-dots just as we did in coloring books when we were young. The downside is that there are few to no pictures that are adult dot-to-dot coloring pages. This could be a hint to people who are artists as well as therapists or nurses who may want to use their talent in creating something new for older adults. Nonetheless, people who use dot-to-dots have to find the sequential numbers (keep these simple depending on the mind functioning of an individual), and connect them. When they are done, they can even paint or color in the picture.

A few other cognitive activities for geriatric patients include music (which also is emotional), table games, word finds, current events, cards, and puzzles. There are companies that are now designing puzzles with adult-level themes, which have big pieces and make a 2- by 5-foot puzzle. S&S Crafts, for example, has a set of three 300-piece puzzles of vintage cafes. Melissa & Doug® has done sealife, rain forest, and solar system 100-piece puzzles that may easily be assembled and cost relatively little. In a mental health setting when working with new admissions, this is a great activity that aids in assessing social skills, length of ability to remain on task, eye–hand skills, and spatial awareness. For three to five people, these puzzles can be completed in 60 to 90 minutes. Given all that, the same puzzle done independently or with just one other individual can be less frustrating for an older adult because it can be finished in a shorter period of time.

Rummy, Skip-bo®, dominoes, and UNO® are games that can be used with their usual rules or the rules adapted for groups that have more difficulty with their memory. It is helpful to have the person count his or her own score in each round; however, keeping track of those scores in each hand/round is not imperative. These same activities can provide knowledge on the social, spatial, and mental functioning of an individual (see Appendix 16C).

A favorite activity with individuals is writing. Poetry is an easy way to teach writing skills by using cinquains, haiku, diamentes, or other simple poem styles. Ingrid Wendt is an Oregon poet who has taught poetry writing at grade levels K–12, and I was able to visualize from her book *Starting With Little Things* how I could improve my use of poetry in therapeutic recreation. Here are a few examples of group poems written in a class this author taught for older adults (see Appendix 16D).

Laughter
Joyful, harmonious
Exercising, healing, relaxing
Remarks, emotions, feelings, jokes
Hurting, cutting, damaging
Bitter, upset
Anger

Chair	Harvest moon above
Blue, large	Crossing over planet large.
Rolling, moving sleeping	Wheat in fields swaying.
Rocking chair soothes baby	
Cradle.	

Regardless of the class, each person can go away with results, some use of language skills, a time to interact with others, and perhaps even a new skill to incorporate into his or her life.

SUMMARY

- Clients and caregivers need to be their own best advocates because all health care workers, medical clinics, and facilities are not created equal.
- Health professionals are human and subject to fatigue, illness, and make errors in judgment.

- Communication breakdowns can be very frustrating and cost time and energy to clarify information.
- Medical records get lost. Faxes and even electronic reports may end up in someone else's chart or simply floating in the ethernet. Every client or caregiver needs to keep copies of medical visits and reports to carry to medical visits (see Appendix 16A).
- The doctor shortage is one indication that clients may no longer rely on the hometown doctor to remember everything about them. Seeing multiple doctors over a series of several visits adds to confusion and further underlines the need for the client or caregiver to keep a record of events, instructions, medication changes, and so on.
- Ideal is not reality and clients and caregivers must be alert to protect themselves. If the client is a resident in a care facility, how can family or friends be assured that the client is receiving all the care agreed upon in the contract? Who makes occasional, unannounced visits to make sure soiled briefs are changed in a timely manner or that the resident has had adequate nutrition for the day?
- RNs are not always on staff for optional living facilities. Many times they work primarily in an administrative role, with very little time to supervise personal caregivers.
- Turnover is high for caregivers for many reasons: low pay, inflexible hours, long work hours, and it's simply very hard work.
- Overworked staff, who may experience lack of adequate supplies for client care may experience moral burnout and moral residue.
- Clients and their personal health manager (family, friend, and/or case manager) need to be empowered to advocate for quality health care. There are tactful ways of addressing concerns, but if it appears that the concerns are not taken seriously, then it may be time to bring in backup and a list of concerns and expectations.
- Recreation therapy offers many health benefits for clients and caregivers.

RESOURCES

Attitude Toward Geriatric Nursing Shortage

http://www.nursetogether.com/attitude-geriatrics-nursing-shortage

Search Terms
- Prestigious work
- Professional pride

Empowering Patients by Kathy Quan, RN, BSN, PHN

http://www.netplaces.com/new-nurse/the-patients/empowering-patients.htm

Search Terms
- How to cope
- What to expect
- What to do

National Association of American Agencies on Aging

http://www.n4a.org

Search Terms
- Advocacy
- Answers on aging

National Center for Assisted Living

http://www.ahcancal.org/ncal/operations/Documents/VRT%20Final%20Report%202011%20Data.pdf

Search Terms
- Staff turnover

REFERENCES

Bonnifield, J., & Cohen, E. (2014). *The empowered patient—10 shocking medical mistakes*. CNN Health–U.S. Edition June 10, 2012. Retrieved May 31, 2014, from http://www.cnn.com/2012/06/09/health/medical-mistakes/index.html

Burkhardt, M. A., & Nathaniel, A. K. (2008). Ethics and issues in contemporary nursing (3rd ed.). Clifton Park, NY : Thomson Delmar Learning.

Cosgrove, D. (2013). *4 Ways to partner with your doctor*. Health Hub from Cleveland Clinic. Retrieved May 31, 2014, from http://health.clevelandclinic.org/2013/07/4-ways-to-partner-with-your-/doctor

Epstein, E., & Delgado, S. (2010). Understanding and addressing moral distress. *Online Journal of Issues in Nursing*, September 30, 2010. Retrieved June 1, 2014, from www.nursingworld.Org/MainMenuCategories/EthicsStandards/courage-and-Distress/Understanding-Moral-Distress.html

Health Resources and Services Administration (HRSA). (2014). *Shortage designation: Health professional shortage areas & medically underserved areas/populations*. U.S. Department of Health and Human Services. Retrieved May 31, 2014, from http://www.hrsa.gov/shortage

Northcutt, J. (2011). *Caregiver turnover impacts care quality*. Care Giver List. Retrieved May 31, 2014, from http://www.caregiverlist.com/SeniorCareNews.aspx/Caregiver%20Turnover%20Impacts%20Care%20Quality

APPENDIX 16A

Make the Most of Your Doctor Appointments

"It seems like the doctor didn't spend even 5 minutes with me before he was off to the next patient!" Have you ever felt this frustration after planning for a doctor visit for several weeks? It's no secret that doctor appointments are tightly scheduled. That is not necessarily the choice of the doctors, but rather it has evolved with the rising cost of health care (and the need to sustain the bottom line). Medical offices are fast-paced, stressful environments for staff and clients. It is important to consider ways we may all help reduce stressful situations.

Our durability as consumers depends on our ability to be flexible and to be our own health care advocate (or the advocate for family members). By accepting the responsibility of an advocate, there is potential for empowerment and to feel more in control of our own health care. I herewith provide you with some tools for the role of advocate.

Be Prepared with the Minimum

I would suggest a notebook or three-ring binder to create a handy portable reference to go with you to doctor appointments: doctor names and contact numbers, preferred pharmacy and contact numbers, insurance information with copy of card, allergies to medications (or other allergies), and blood type.

Always provide a current list of medications being taken (or bring all the medications to the appointment for review). Recent trips to immediate care or a specialist may generate a report for your doctor, but your current list of medications is not updated from those reports. Your primary doctor depends on you to keep track of new medications or dose changes made outside of his or her office. Include the following: *dosage* information includes *strength* of the medication (i.e., mg, g, mcg, unit); *amount* (i.e., 2 mg, 1 g, 40 mcg, 1 unit); and *frequency* (i.e., twice a day, once a day, every 12 hours, or once a week).

Most providers (especially new ones) will want a brief medical and surgical history. Keep this list in your notebook with diagnosis, procedures, facility where performed, and approximate dates.

Helpful Steps

1. Have a list of your medical diagnoses; that is, high blood pressure, low thyroid, or arthritis.
2. Keep a list of questions and concerns that you want to discuss with the doctor.
   - You know time is at a premium and usually there is only time to address one concern. If you know in advance that one appointment slot will not provide enough time, request a longer appointment. This will reduce pressure on you and the doctor. It will help prevent running into someone else's appointment time.
   - We all know how it feels to wait past our scheduled appointment. Sadly, it is perceived as "the doctor is behind" rather than understanding that many patients hope to cover "just one more thing" in their allotted time. Yes, a longer appointment time will increase the fee, but it will save you another trip to discuss more concerns.
3. When scheduling an appointment, calculate 10 minutes per primary concern (add 5–10 minutes per secondary concern). If you cannot get a longer appointment on short notice, be prepared to make another appointment. We know that the geriatric population is increasing, which often means more complex health concerns. No doctor can address multiple concerns in 10 minutes without running over time.

4. Expect the unexpected. Here's where some flexibility comes into the story. No matter how well prepared you are, sometimes things happen and you wind up waiting. Having worked in the back office in clinical settings for many years, I know all about the unexpected. I learned to *space* my personal appointments by an hour or more so that I do not risk running late for the second one. I *report* to my appointment 15 minutes early. If all patients arrive right at appointment time, this delays the check-in process and creates a domino effect against all the following appointments (delay to be roomed, delayed start to appointment). I *expect* that there will be a wait (if there isn't, I am delightfully surprised). I am *prepared* for a wait with a bottle of water, a granola bar, a book, letter-writing material, or needlework. By being prepared for a wait, I know my blood pressure will not be sky-high by the time I get into the examination room.
5. Help reduce your stress and the stress of others by initiating a friendly chat with someone else who is waiting. Just getting started is the big hurdle, but take the initiative and comment about the weather. From there, perhaps inquire how long the person has lived in this area. It gets easier from there. You will be amazed how a friendly conversation can ease tension for everyone in the waiting area (and you just might find a new friend or a lost relative).

SUMMARY

- With medical appointment time at a premium, it is important that we learn how to advocate for ourselves.
- An important part of advocacy is that we know how the current system works so that we can plan strategically.
- Being organized with our own health information will help improve two-way communication between us and our health care providers.

- Schedule enough appointment time to discuss your concerns. Remember, in spite of the best-laid plans, the unexpected happens. When you check in you might inquire if the doctor is on time. If he is not, make a decision to reschedule or wait.
- Be prepared for a wait by thinking of your own comfort (water, snack, book, neck pillow for a nap).

Source: Originally printed in "The Chimes" newsletter, by Brenda L. Bonham Howe, 2010, First United Methodist Church, Bend, Oregon.

APPENDIX 16B

Creative Expression in Therapeutic Recreation

Activity	Benefit
Woodworking 　Pre-cut and/or assembled	Eye–hand coordination through sanding and gluing Social interaction with others in group Independence in selection of paints/colors Cognitive in following instructions
Painting/Drawing	Eye–hand coordination Social interaction with others in group Self-expression Emotional 　• Self-pride when task is completed 　• Recall of past experiences
Beadwork/Jewelry Making	Eye–hand coordination Self-expression Cognitive in following instructions Self-expression 　• Picking colors 　• Choosing style Emotional 　• Self-pride when task is completed 　• Recall of past experiences
Sewing/Knitting/Crocheting	Eye–hand coordination Hand exercise Self-expression 　• Picking patterns 　• Choosing colors 　• Choosing fabric/yarns

Activity	Benefit

	Social interaction
	    • Choosing to give completed work to someone
	    • Talking to group about selection
	Recall of past

Model Making	Eye–hand coordination
	Hand exercise
	Cognitive in following instructions
	Self-expression
	    • Choosing style
	    • Choosing colors to paint
	Recall of past experiences
	Social Interaction
	    • Choosing to give completed work to someone
	    • Talking to group about selection

Gardening
  Raised beds/planters
    pots gardens
	Use of hands
	Recall of past
	Independence: Ability to select
	Responsibility in continued care of garden/plant
	Social interaction/interdependence
	Texture and color identification
	Scent identification

APPENDIX 16C

Cognitive Activities for the Aging Population

Activity	Benefits
Cards	
Rummy	Recall
	Social interaction/cooperativeness
	Counting/math skills
	Sequencing
	Number identification
UNO	Recall
	Color identification
	Number identification
	Sequencing
	Ability to follow directions
	Social interactions/cooperativeness
Skip-Bo	Recall
	Number identification
	Counting/math skills
	Sequencing
	Ability to follow directions
	Social interactions/cooperativeness
Table Games	
Dominoes (there are several different games of dominoes, also referred to as "bones" in the African American culture; Mexican Train is another type of domino game)	Number/color matching of dots
	Ability to count in fives/math skills
	Ability to follow directions
	Sequencing

Activity	Benefits
Rummy Kube (similar to the card game)	Recall Social interaction/cooperativeness Counting Sequencing Number identification
Scrabble and Upwords	Spelling skills Social interactions/cooperative Ability to follow rules Mathematic skills
Dancing Line dancing	Eye–hand coordination Memory skills Reminiscence
Writing Journaling	Reminiscence Life review Work on acceptance of current functioning
Story writing	Sequencing Reminiscence Creativity
Poetry writing	Creativity Focusing on life experiences Awareness of nature/people/events Ability to learn/recall poetry styles Social skills (sometimes work as a group to create a poem)
Puzzles Jigsaw puzzles (can be extra large pieces; always should be age appropriate)	Spacial awareness Cooperation with others Eye–hand coordination Attention span Aware of photos within the puzzle

APPENDIX 16D

Emotional and Social Therapeutic Recreation Activities

Music and Writing	Benefits
Drumming	Self-identity (sets own rhythm or has own role depending on the type of rhythm instrument)
	Becomes part of a group/interreliability
	Rhythm (all life has rhythm)
	Does not require previous experience
	Can be used with all disabilities (paddle drums can be secured to the chair of someone who has motor disabilities or has had a stroke)
Singing	
Choir	Cognitive
	• Recall of learning music notes
	Social interaction
	Part of a group
	Performing/sharing with others
	Recall of past music experiences
Music group	Cognitive
	• Recall music from earlier life experience
	• Remembering life experiences
	Social interaction
Spiritual Groups (respect required for all faiths/beliefs)	Allow expression of faith or belief
	Guided memories of faith experiences
	Social interaction/connection with others with similar experiences or beliefs
	Self-expression about future fears/beliefs

Music and Writing	Benefits
Poetry Writing/Writing	Cognitive recall of present or past (family, experiences, places she or he has been to, leisure/recreation interests)
	Cognitive functioning in learning styles of writing
	Self-identity
	Self-expression
	Means of learning individual's interests
	Social interaction (when reading his or her poem or sharing it in written form)
Reading	
Folktales	Recall of past
Classics	• Sparks discussion of past experiences
Westerns	• Relates to positive/negative experiences and how to resolve them
Life stories of people with similar diseases	Reality orientation
Spiritual	Emotional
	• Story brings joy/sadness
Chimes	Use of eye–hand coordination
	Arm exercise
	Cognitive by reading letters that match individual chime
	Recall
	• Letter/note of chime
	• Music known from past
	Emotional
	Social interdependence to play a musical piece

Index

activity theory, 69
acute hearing loss, 79
age-related memory loss, 86
aging and physical changes
    theoretical perspectives on,
        57–73, *See also* theories on
        aging
age-related hearing loss
    (ARHL), 79
allostatic load, 65–66
Alzheimer's disease (AD), 88
    caregivers, 88–89, 248
    data on, 248
    and memory care, 247–252
    residential care transformation
        into memory care, 247–248
American College of Physicians
    (ACP), 113
American Foot Care Association
    (AFCA), 84
American Hospital Association
    (AHA), 113
American Medical Association
    (AMA), 113

American Nurses Association
    (ANA), 113
American Psychiatric Association
    (APA), 5
anointing of the sick, 28
assisted living/assisted-living
    facilities (ALFs), 227–236
    activities, 229
    amenities, 228–229
    funding, 235
    licensure/regulatory agencies,
        234
    safety, 229–230
    staff members, 230–232
    staffing requirements, 232
    staff-to-resident ratio, 233–234
    training, 232–233
Assisted Living Facilities
    Organization (ALFO),
    230
Assisted Living Federation of
    America (ALFA), 233–234
associate degree nurses (ADN),
    242–243

baccalaureate degree nurses (BSNs), 242
biological theories of aging, 58
burden of care
  factors increasing, 3
Bureau of Indian Affairs (BIA), 36–37
burnout, 6, 266
Bush, George W., 6

caregivers, 5–6
  burnout, 6, 266
caregiving
  mental health and, 5–6
Catholicism, 25–28
Centers for Disease Control and Prevention (CDC), 81, 114
Centers for Medicare and Medicaid Services (CMS), 116, 199
certified nursing assistant (CNA), 221, 232–233, 242–243
certified therapeutic recreation specialist (CTRS), 269
clinical educator, 191–192
Codman, Ernest, 119–120
cognitive activities, 282–283
  for geriatric patients, 271–272
Communion, 27
community health clinics, 256
Conditions for Coverage (CfCs), Medicare, 117, 119
Conditions of Participation (CoPs), Medicare, 117, 119
continuity theory, 68
cross-linked model of aging, 63–64
cultural domain and health care delivery, 22

Culturally and Linguistically Appropriate Services (CLAS), 12, 22
culturally appropriate services standards, 12–13
Curanderismo, 30
curanderos, 31
current home care organizations, 114

Dawes Allotment Act of 1887, 37
day care, 103–104
deeming, 117
Department of Health and Human Services (DHHS), 116
diagnosis-related groups (DRGs), 112
discrimination, 15
disengagement theory, 68–69
doctor deficit, 263
doctor of podiatric medicine (DPM), 84

ego transcendence versus ego preoccupation, 72
end-of-life (EOL) care, 32, 49–50, 181
  hospice nurse in, 211–214
end-stage renal disease (ESRD), 116
Erikson's stage of integrity versus despair, 70
error theories, 58, 62–67
  allostatic load, 65–66
  cross-link, 63–64
  free radicals, 64–65
  metabolic syndrome, 66–67
  somatic mutations, 63
  wear and tear, 65
ethical burnout, 266
ethical responsibilities, 15–16
  organizational awareness, 15–16
ethnocentrism, 14

Eucharist, 27
Evangelical Protestantism, 28–29
Extreme Unction, 28

family model, Hispanics, 24
federal Medicare expenditure, 111
financially compromised
   additional community health resources for, 255–258
food in Hispanic culture, 32
foot care RN (FCRN), 192–193
foot health
   and aging, 82
   intervention, 84–85
footwear
   as an environmental risk factor, 83
   styles of, 84
free radicals, 64
funding, 221
   and financial issues, 204
fungal affected nails, 83

Garbach, Lidia, 270
gender role, Hispanic population, 25
geriatric clients, 4–5, 6
geriatric population, recreation therapy for, 268–272
grief process, 3
group homes, 104–105

Havighurst, Robert, 69
Hayflick, Leonard, 59
Hayflick limit, 59
health belief model (HBM), 22–24
health care access, 15
health care and health issues, attitudes about, 29, *See also* indigenous/folk healing practices

health care conflict, 13–14
health care delivery
   conflicts, 13–14
   cultural considerations, 11
   cultural domains, 21–50
   ethical responsibilities, 15–16
   interpreter validation, 12–13
   minority growth, 11
   psychosocial barriers to, 14
   racism, 14–15
health nurse, 220
hearing loss
   intervention of, 80
hearing problems and aging, 79
Henderson, Virginia, 179–180
Hispanics, 24–34
   attitudes about health issues, 29–32
   Catholicism, 25
   family model, 24
   gender role in health care, 25
   health and illness in, 24
   health care information, limitations in, 33–34
   language barriers in, 32–33
   potential problems and solutions, 32–34
   primary health care providers lacking among, 33
   religious or spiritual needs and health, 25–29
home care
   agencies, categories of, 114
   Medicare and Medicaid documentation, 132–178
   nursing practice, definition of, 112–114
   in United States, 111
home health, what is provided by Medicare, 116–120

home health aide (HHA), 102,
    123–124, 184
home health nursing practice
    definition of, 112–114
    documentation, 185
    focuses of, 113
home health nursing supervisor,
    193–194
home health program coordinator
    (HHPC), 194–195
home health services
    job descriptions, 123–128
    Medicare approved, 116–120
    organizations, 114–116
    qualifications for, 120–121
    skilled medical care, 120–121
    in the United States, 111–114
home health team members
    services provided by, 121–122
home safety inspection, 98–99
home-style adult safety and
    socialization options, 97
home-style options
    amenities, 105
    group homes, 104–105
    in-home caregiver options, 100
    licensure requirements, 104
    private caregiver, 101
    private duty caregivers, 101–102
    private duty home care
        agencies, 101
    remodel, 99–100
    significance of, 97–98
    staff and training, 103, 106
home to community, 4–5
hospice care, 200–201
    funding and financial issues, 204
    services from, 201
hospice nurses, 211
    as students of human nature, 213

hospice services, documents
    requirement, 132–178
    ADL/IADL, 160–166
    cardiac status, 154–155
    care management, 169–172
    clinical record items, 135–136
    data items collected, 175–178
    elimination status, 155–156
    emergent care, 174–175
    home health patient tracking
        sheet, 132–133
    integumentary status, 148–153
    living arrangements, 145–146
    medications, 166–169
    neuro/emotional/behavioral
        status, 156–160
    outcome and assessment
        information set, 134–135
    patient history and diagnoses,
        136–145
    respiratory status, 154
    sensory status, 146–148
    therapy need and plan of care,
        172–174
hospice registered nurse (RN), 203
hospice services, 199–200
    initiation, 202
    skilled nurse competency
        requirements for, 211–212
    start of hospice, 199
hospital-based home health
    agencies, 115
hypothalamus–pituitary–adrenal
    feedback loop (HPA axis), 61–62

independent living, 217
    activities, 218
    amenities, 217–218
    costs associated with, 221
    definition of, 217

education requirements, 220
funding, 221
health nurse, 220
licensure/regulatory
   agencies, 221–222
safety, 219
scope of practice, 219, 220
staff members, 219, 220
Indian Health Services (IHS), 40
Indian Removal Act (1830), 36
indigenous/folk healing
   practices, 30–31
infection control nurse (ICN),
   195–196
in-home caregiver options, 100
intake RN, 182–183
interdisciplinary team (IDT) for
   hospice care, 200–201
internal revenue service (IRS), 115
*The International Council of Nurses
   Code of Ethics 2012 (ICNC)*, 15,
   22, 267
International Medical Interpreters
   Association (IMIA), 13
interpreter validation, 12–13

language assistance, 12–14
licensed practical nurse (LPN),
   102, 231, 233, 242
licensed vocational nurse (LVN),
   102, 231, 242
licensing for private duty home
   care, 102–103
licensure, 104, 105–106
licensure/regulatory agencies,
   221–222, 234
life course theory, 67–68
life span increase, 1
linguistically appropriate services
   standards, 12

long-term care (LTC), 241–245
   definition, 241
   education requirements, 242–243
   funding, 244
   licensure/regulatory agencies, 244
   scope of practice, 242–243
   staff members, 242–243
Lower Extremity Amputation
   Prevention (LEAP), 84

Medicaid programs, 116
medical social worker, 127–128
Medicare, 111, 116, 118, 234–235
   conditions of participation, 117, 119
Medicare coverage, 117–118, 120
Medicare hospice benefit, 200
   eligibility conditions for, 200
memory care
   client-centered care, 250–251
   philosophy of, 249–251
   residential care transformation
      into, 247–248
memory loss
   and aging, 86
   interventions for, 87–88
   symptoms of, 86–87
mental changes of aging, 77
mental health
   and caregiving, 5–6
metabolic syndrome, 66–67
minority growth, 11
Montessori, Maria, 249–250
moral burnout, 266
musculoskeletal changes
   and aging, 80–82
   interventions for, 81–82

nail care, 85
National Association of Home
   Care (NAHC), 113

National Board of Certification
    for Medical Interpreters
    (NBCMI), 13
National Board for Certification of
    Hospice and Palliative Care
    Nurses (NBCHPN), 214
National CLAS Standards,
    12–13, 22
National Council on Interpreting
    in Health Care (NCIHC), 13
National Hospice and Palliative
    Care Organization (NHPCO),
    204–205, 208, 213–215
Native Americans
    assimilation and allotment
        period, 37–38
    beliefs and values, 42–44
    Bureau of Indian Affairs (BIA), 37
    care considerations among, 48–50
    communication among, 44–45
    Dawes Allotment Act, 37
    early health concerns, 41
    healing traditions among, 47–48
    health and illness among,
        34–35, 47
    health care needs, 41–42
    historical background, 35–40
    Indian Health Care
        Improvement Act, 39
    Indian Health Services (IHS), 38
    Indian Removal Act (1830), 36
    Indian Self-Determination and
        Education Assistance Act, 39
    nonverbal communication
        among, 45
    reservation period, 36–37
    self-determination period, 39
    shifting to chronic diseases, 41–42
    spiritual beliefs among, 45–47
    termination period, 38–39
    treaty period, 36
nonmedical caregivers, 2
Northwest Portland Area Indian
    Health Board [NPAIHB], 40
nurse competency requirements
    basic care components, 180
    for home health services, 179
    job descriptions, 182
    nursing code of ethics, 15, 22, 267
    position qualifications, 182
    RN expectations, 182
    skills, 181
nursing assistant registered
    (NAR), 243
nursing shortage, 6–7

occupational therapist, 126
Office of Management and Budget
    (OMB), 132
official home care agencies, 114–115
older adulthood, Peck's stages of,
    71–72
OMB. *See* Office of Management
    and Budget (OMB)
onychomycosis (toenail fungus), 83
orichas, 30
Outcome and Assessment
    Instrument Set (OASIS), 122

palliative care, 204–205
Pardo, Ann, 270
parish nurses, 257
Peck, Robert, 71
Peck's stages of older adulthood,
    71–72
personal care assistant (PCA), 102,
    220–221
personal care assistant versus
    certified nursing assistant,
    220–221

personal construct psychology
  (PCP), 3
personal touch from hospice
  nurse, 212
philosophy in memory care,
  Montessori's system of,
  249–250
physical and mental changes of
  aging, 77
physical changes associated with
  aging, 78–80
  hearing problems, 79
  vision, 78–79
physical therapist, 125
pipe ceremonies, 47, 48
pituitary gland, 61–62
podiatrist, 84
prejudice, 14
primary care provider
  (PCP), 181
privacy among Hispanics, 31–32
private caregiver, 101
private duty caregivers 101–102
private duty home care
  agencies, 101
  licensing for, 102–103
private nonprofit agencies, 115
programmed theories, 58–62
  Hayflick limit, 59–60
  immunological, 60–61
  neuroendocrine, 61–62
promotoras, 33–34
proprietary agencies, 115–116
psychosocial barriers
  to successful health care
  delivery, 14
psychosocial–cultural health, 1–7
  growing old, 3–4
  home to community, 4–5
  psychosocial impact, 2–3

psychosocial theories of aging,
  67–72, *See also* activity
  theory; continuity theory;
  disengagement theory; life
  course theory

quality coordinator (QC), 196–197

racism, 14–15
radio babies, 97
reconciliation, 27
recreation therapy
  cognitive activities, 271
  creative expression, 280–281
  emotional and social
    therapeutic recreation
    activities, 284
  games, 271
  for geriatric population,
    268–272
  physical exercise, 269
  swimming, 269
  yoga, 270
Reagan, Ronald, 111
registered dietician, 128
registered nurse (RN), 100, 123, 179,
  182–183, 242–243
  admissions, 185–186
  essential job functions, 183–185
  foot care RN, 192–193
  job description, 183, 185
  position qualifications, 191
  RN case manager, 187
  RN–on call, 186–187
  RN–tele-health co-ordinator, 188
  RN–triage, 189–190
  wound, ostomy, continence
    nurse (WOCN), 190–191
regulatory agencies, 116–120
rehabilitation, 81–82

religious or spiritual needs of Hispanics and health, 25–29
residential care facilities (RCFs), 228
    types, 228
residential care transformation into memory care, 247–248
respeto, 29–30
Resumption of Care (ROC), 132, 134–136
retirement communities, 217–218
ROC. *See* Resumption of Care (ROC)

sacramentals, 27
sacraments, 27
safety, 229–230
safety inspectors, 98–100
Santeria, 30
santero, 30
scapular, 27
self-advocacy
    doctor deficit, 263
    empowering the inner advocate, 267
    human side of professionals, 262
    moral and ethical burnout, 266
    moral residue, 266–267
    need for, 261
    nurse, myth of, 264–265
    positive relief, 267–268
    staff retention, 265–266
    taking charge of medical records, 262–263
shared responsibilities, 121–122
skilled medical care, 120–121
somatic mutations, 63
speech therapist, 126–127
spirituality among Native Americans, 45–47

staff members
    scope of practice, and education requirements, 220
staff retention, 265–266
start of hospice, 199–200
State Children's Health Insurance Program (SCHIP), 117
stereotyping, 14
sweat ceremonies, 46, 47–48

teacher caregivers, 251
tele-health coordinator, 188
The Joint Commission (TJC), 117, 119–120
theories on aging, 57–69
    activity theory, 69
    biological theories of aging, 58
    continuity theory, 68
    disengagement theory, 68–69
    error theories, 62–67
    life course theory, 67–68
    programmed theories, 58–62
    psychosocial theories, 67–72
total parenteral nutrition (TPN), 143

United States, home care in, 111–114

vision changes and aging, 78
vision loss
    intervention of, 78–79
voluntary agencies, 115

wear and tear and aging, 65
Wendt, Ingrid, 272
Westberg, Granger, 257
wound, ostomy, continence nurse (WOCN), 190–191